RADIANT WOMAN

Every Woman's Guide to Health, Healing and Rejuvenation

By

Maggie Erotokritou

ISBN: 1-4107-0181-6 (e-book)
ISBN: 1-4107-0182-4 (Paperback)

This book is printed on acid free paper.

1stBooks – rev 1/17/03

The contents of this book are for information only and are not intended to be a substitute for taking proper medical advice from a doctor or health practitioner when needed. The author has attempted to give a profound understanding of the topics discussed and to ensure accuracy and completeness of any information given to the best of her personal knowledge and expertise. Any use of the information set forth herein is entirely at the reader's discretion. The author and publisher are not responsible for any adverse effects or consequences resulting from the ideas given in this book. Readers should use their own judgment or consult a holistic medical expert or their personal physician for individual problems.

To all those who have guided, inspired and supported me on my journey and to all the wonderful women known and unknown who share the journey with me.

Contents

Introduction

Radiant women have an inner beauty that stands out. They are not necessarily beautiful in the traditional way, because of their outer looks, facial features, body shape or size. It is their presence that comes forth, their warmth, their joy and their way of being that makes them attractive. A radiant woman glows, her eyes sparkle and her smile dazzles. She radiates a blissful aura, her energy is powerful and centered and she is clear and positive. A radiant woman knows how to nurture and take care of herself. She takes responsibility for her health and well-being, listens to her body and pays attention to how she feels and acts accordingly.

The emphasis of this book is on creating radiant health, and healing whatever stands in the way. Radiant health is more than just feeling physically good or being disease free, it is about being filled with energy, vitality and joy, being emotionally stable and having a mental outlook that will constantly expand your horizons. Your energy level is a measure of how you feel. In order to have enough energy to do what you want to do and to fully express your creative inspiration, you have to pay attention to the physical, emotional, mental and spiritual aspects of yourself. If any part is ignored, this will create an imbalance.

After many years of working with women in the fields of therapy and different healing systems including Ayurveda, managing the Surya Health and Healing Centre in Cyprus and co-ordinating the international Women's Spiritual Network, I gained a lot of insights into the needs of women in respect to the fields of health and healing. Again and again, I would hear the same questions and cries for help and understanding and requests for more knowledge. There was so much to share but never enough time to give it. It was out of these desires, needs and requests that this book was born.

Many of the gems that it contains are based upon my knowledge and training as an Ayurvedic health consultant. It is not however primarily a book on Ayurveda, it is based upon a deep exploration into different healing modalities. It is a practical book, which enables the reader to take responsibility for their own health and healing and to open up new avenues and possibilities for healing. This book is not meant to be a replacement for medical treatment; it is a complimentary approach to health care especially in the prevention of disease and goes beyond that to include the possibility of regeneration and rejuvenation. It is full of many life-enhancing ideas, which are easily put into practise.

By directing your attention towards maintaining radiant health, it will also allow your innate wisdom to come forth and support the process. Many women have lost their intuitive knowingness; they have forgotten how to listen to the whispers of their inner wisdom, this book will help you regain that wisdom. Health and healing go hand in hand. By creating new, supportive and healthier habits, you can change the way you feel and this will be reflected outwardly. When our health improves, then both emotional and physical healing can take place and when we heal our emotional wounds and traumas, we feel more inclined to look after our health.

Each of us has the potential to become a radiant woman and to enjoy life to the full with passion and joy. It has nothing to do with age; it is about how you feel inside. You have to ignite the flame of life within and to keep it burning brightly until the last breath passes out of the body. In order to do this, you have to nurture yourself well and become aware of anything that prevents this from happening and then an amazing metamorphosis can take place.

PART 1

HEALTH, OUR MOST PRECIOUS GIFT

Maggie Erotokritou

1 – RADIANT HEALTH

Our health is the most precious gift we have and it needs to be treasured. Radiant health depends upon many factors; the constitution you were born with, your genes, body type, lifestyle factors, hormones, metabolism, psychological health, mental attitude, monthly cycles, environmental factors and planetary influences.

A major factor of radiant health lies in creating balance between the overall function and maintenance of the body and the co-ordination of the different body systems and organs and the full understanding of the effect of the mind upon the body and visa versa. Besides paying attention to our physical needs, we also need to maintain our psychological balance by learning how to efficiently handle stress and keep stress levels to a minimum. Everyone wants to be able to work at a peak performance level and to be as creative and productive as possible, this requires learning how to pace oneself in the right way and developing the right attitude to whatever is occurring in the moment.

Being radiant is much more than just being healthy, it is a state of being where you are filled with so much energy and vitality that it surges through your whole being and extends outwards to inspire others. When the life force energy flows abundantly through every channel of the body, the energy level is high and this enables one to transcend the normal process of ageing.

Choosing to take personal responsibility for your health is empowering because it opens you to many new possibilities that you may not have previously considered and encourages you to make better choices regarding your health. Radiant health is an essential key to youthfulness, which is not to do with your chronological age but how you feel inside and that depends upon how well you nurture and look after yourself. In living a lifestyle that is totally supportive of your well-being, you can maintain radiant health throughout your life.

Ayurvedic Wisdom

Ayurveda is an ancient, natural health care system from India. Ayur means life and Veda means knowledge. It is known as the science of life and longevity, which was recorded in the ancient Vedic texts and is thousands of years old. Ayurveda provides a wealth of knowledge on living harmoniously and recreating balance through using natural methods of healing. Ayurveda was brought to the West by different Indian sages and doctors, the most well known being Maharishi Mahesh Yogi who worked with Dr. Deepak Chopra to create a system that was accessible and comprehensible and could easily be incorporated into the western way of life. I was very privileged to be one of the first people to be trained in this system. My training in Maharishi Ayurveda was one of the greatest gifts of my life and it opened me to a completely new approach to health and healing.

Ayurveda places emphasis on living in accordance with natural law in order to restore harmony and balance and enjoy radiant health. Correct diet, a sattvic lifestyle and the right amount of sleep are considered to be the fundamental pillars of well-being. When the mind, body, senses and emotions work harmoniously together, then the natural intelligence of the body is awakened and healing can take place. It is said that where there is balance and flow, disease cannot flourish, but where there is stagnation, blockage or imbalance, disease can manifest. In Ayurveda, the focus is always on health and maintaining a state of equilibrium and looking at ways to bring the person back to balance and a state of ease, rather than dis-ease.

For example if there is too much fire or heat in the body, it should be cooled, if there is not enough fire, it must be ignited and stoked, if there is not enough moisture it must be added, too much moisture needs to be dried. If movement is too slow it must be increased, if there is too much activity, which causes irritation, it must be reduced. Energy blockages need to be released and stagnant energy dispersed and redirected to other parts of the body.

Ayurveda is a holistic approach that takes everything into consideration; it looks at the whole person, rather than the parts, as well as a person's lifestyle including the climate and environment they live in. An Ayurvedic physician or consultant can tell a lot about a person just by looking at them. The way a person stands, their speech, the way they express themselves, their face, eyes, skin and their particular smell, all tell a part of their story. Ayurveda is unique in its approach to different body types and makes recommendations accordingly. It takes deep sensitivity and development on the part of the practitioner to develop the ability to read the pulse and discern what a person needs. This ability is enhanced through many years of practice of meditation.

Diagnosis and personal recommendations are made through pulse diagnosis and through evaluating a person's basic constitution and lifestyle and current and past imbalances. It is believed that there is no one treatment for everyone because each person is so unique; therefore consequently the recommendations will vary from person to person. Ayurveda is a vast and complex system, which is not easily understood. It has become more popular in the West over the last fifteen to twenty years, especially amongst those who seek a more natural and holistic way of living and are interested to take responsibility for their own health and healing.

Ayurveda believes that the root of illness lies in the mind and stems from wrong thinking, which results in incorrect behaviour and destructive habits, which create imbalances between the mind, body and the senses. Right lifestyle, diet, Yoga, meditation and spiritual practices help activate the body's natural intelligence and ability to heal. Everything we do should be enjoyable. When we create this inner state of joy and harmony, we create what is known as a sattvic state and this produces bliss hormones known as ojas.

Ayurveda deeply honours and reveres women, it understands that women need to be treated in a special way and that their bodies function differently from men, especially their nervous and hormonal systems. A lot of attention is given to help women re-establish and maintain their natural balance and there are specific herbs, teas and oils, especially for women.

Ayurveda is an exciting science, which is continuously evolving. It encompasses all areas of life including the study of the mind and consciousness. Ayurveda believes that many problems arise from a lack of consciousness and unwise choices, which are made through a lack of clarity. When our consciousness expands and the mind is open and unlimited, we naturally move in the direction of radiant health, personal growth and purposeful living.

Body Types

Ayurveda is unique in its holistic approach to different body types and classifies them into ten categories. Recommendations for healing and therapy always take into account a person's body type. Our body type consists of our basic constitution, genetic make up and the uniqueness of our DNA coding, which influence the specific functioning of the mind and body. No one is exactly the same as anyone else. We may have similar physical structures including a brain, a skeleton, the same organs and bodily systems but each of us looks, feels and behaves differently. We are different shapes and sizes, have different skin colours and live in different countries with different climates, customs and lifestyles. All of these add to our uniqueness. Yet often the medical profession would have us believe that we are all the same and tries to categorize and treat us in this way. Because of our uniqueness, we naturally respond differently and have different desires and preferences.

Ayurveda categorizes the ten specific body types according to the influence of the three doshas, vata, pitta and kapha. These are the three fundamental principles, which govern all the actions of the mind and body. Vata is dominated by air and governs movement, breathing, circulation and elimination. Pitta is dominated by fire and governs digestion, metabolism and processing. Kapha is dominated by earth and water and governs structure and fluid balance. We have all three doshas present in us in varying degrees but one or two doshas may be more dominant or active.

For example, a person could be a vata/pitta combination, or a pitta/vata, or pitta/kapha etc. The most prominent dosha is placed first. Reading Ayurvedic books may help you determine your basic constitution or to recognize your natural tendencies, but to determine your imbalances and re-establish the balance of all three doshas requires a deeper level of experience and understanding.

Some people are born with a strong constitution and therefore have the advantage of a strong immune system. These people seem to be able to eat anything or live any sort of lifestyle without easily going off balance. This is however deceptive, for even people with a strong constitution need to take care otherwise at some point in life usually around middle age or even later, the results of undesirable habits become apparent. Whereas people with a weaker constitution may appear to be at a disadvantage because their body may react quicker to any imbalances but this can also be seen as advantageous because their body gives them earlier messages to pay attention in order to restore balance. It is easier to restore smaller imbalances rather than major ones. We have all heard stories of people who appeared to be fine and healthy suddenly having a heart attack or becoming very ill. This was not a sudden occurrence, the imbalances had probably been manifesting slowly in the body for a period of twenty or thirty years until it eventually reached a crisis point. For this reason prevention is always better than cure and the whole approach of Ayurveda is to enhance health so that imbalances and disease cannot have the opportunity to take hold.

Different body types naturally have certain preferences. For example, a vata dominant body type tends to feel the cold more and therefore prefers hot drinks and food and loves hot climates. Whereas a pitta dominant body type has a lot of heat in the body and prefers cooling drinks and foods and dislikes hot climates. This explains why you might see two people walking down the street; one is a vata person, dressed warmly wearing trousers, a jacket and a shawl, whereas the other is a pitta person wearing a tea shirt and shorts. Vata people are usually thin and can eat as much as they like without putting on weight, kapha people say they only have to look at food and they put on weight, they are also the ones who have difficulty losing weight. Pitta people have a tendency towards allergies and have to be more careful of what they eat. Vata people can get anxious when they are imbalanced, pitta can have a sharp tongue and may be prone to anger whereas kapha people tend to take things more in their stride and rarely get upset.

Balanced vata tends to be very enthusiastic and vibrant, imbalanced vata can be anxious, restless and prone to sleep problems. Balanced pitta enjoys challenges, has a strong, clear mind and is articulate. Imbalanced Pitta can be irritable and impatient, angry or demanding. Kapha is steady and relaxed and has good stamina; imbalanced kapha likes to oversleep, becomes lethargic, loses motivation and doesn't like to exercise. These are just a few of the principles that apply to the different body types. No body type is better than another; it is always a question of balancing the different aspects of ourselves.

Taking responsibility for your health

Our health is so precious yet often we take it for granted until we get sick or feel unwell. Taking responsibility for your health is empowering. As you become more aware of what increases or decreases your vitality and what makes you feel good and what doesn't, you will want to become more health conscious and make better life enhancing choices rather than those which weaken or debilitate. Most imbalances and diseases begin with a decrease in energy or a block in the energy channels. By monitoring your energy level and noticing the fluctuations, what influences it, what gives you energy, what drains it and why you feel different on certain days, you will want to make changes that prevent energy drains. Gradually you will also notice what specific situations or people drain your energy and choose to avoid them.

Radiant health encompasses many things; the following list gives a perspective of what good health is. You may like to add some of your own ideas to the list and tick and give priority to what needs attention.

Radiant health is:

- Feeling really good within one's self, physically, mentally and psychologically.
- Having enough energy and vitality to be able to lead the lifestyle that you choose, enabling you to be active, dynamic and creative.
- Being harmonious and peaceful within oneself and with others.
- Having emotional stability and balance so as to be able to cope with the daily pressures of life without allowing them to have an adverse effect and knowing how to efficiently deal with stress when it occurs.
- For all the body systems, organs and glands to be functioning at the highest possible performance level, especially the processes of circulation, assimilation, digestion and elimination. This is essential for regeneration and rejuvenation.
- To be pain free and flexible regardless of age.
- To have a crystal clear and creative mind.
- To have a good memory both long-term and short-term.
- Being super positive at all times, remembering that our thoughts affect our emotions and body and therefore our health.
- When there is a problem, trying to find the root cause through self-reflection or by exploring different resources rather than seeking a quick, temporary fix.

A Holistic Viewpoint

Thinking holistically means seeing the bigger picture, getting a wider perspective and taking everything into account. There is so much conflicting information on health nowadays, different schools of thought have different ideas and this causes confusion. The trouble stems from the fact that most systems do not take into account personal differences and body types. This means that what works really well for one person may not work for another.

For example, one school of thought may recommend all raw foods, which is fine providing you have a lot of heat in your body, live in a warm climate and have a strong digestion. However, if you are a vata body type, which feels the cold, you will not be happy with only raw food, which does not generate enough heat in your body, this would be even worse if you also live in a cold climate. If your digestion is weak or there are intestinal problems, raw food although considered purifying is hard to digest and could make the problem worse.

If you live in a hot climate, naturally you would want more cooling foods. So your lifestyle, where you live and the climate make a difference to what foods you choose to eat. I teach a lot of Yoga and give rebirthing and healing sessions, so for my work I need to eat regularly but lightly. Living in Cyprus, the summers are very hot so it suits my body type and lifestyle to drink lots of fresh juices and to eat lots of salads, but in the winter when it cools down, I need lots of hot and nourishing foods. A builder or someone who does a lot of physical work needs more substantial food in the morning, they would not be able to exist just on fruit juice for breakfast but would benefit more from a nourishing bowl of porridge. You have to be aware of your needs at the present time and be flexible and adapt according to the circumstances. The advice that is given in the book on diet is therefore general and not intended to replace personal recommendations but it will point you in the direction on living a more conscious and healthy lifestyle.

Whenever we go through a seasonal change, the body also goes through a transition too. It is therefore recommended during these times to take extra care of your health and you may find that you need more rest and sleep. During seasonal changes, it is also beneficial to detoxify in order to help the body make the necessary adjustments and release any toxic build up that have accumulated from the previous season. This is also a good time to have reflexology or healing sessions to boost your immune system.

All the body systems are designed to work holistically together, when one system breaks down, all the other systems are affected too, nothing works in isolation. Everything in the body is governed by the brain, which acts like a master computer linking all the different systems together and monitoring everything that is happening in the body. Messages are sent through the nervous system, which is an intricate and sophisticated network, to inform each part of the body what is going on elsewhere. When something goes wrong in one part of the body, all the other parts try to support and correct the problem.

Everything we have ever experienced is recorded in the DNA, all our joys, our highs and lows, traumas and fears. If we listen to the deep intelligence of the body, it will guide us on how to heal the body and tell us what is good for us and what is not. Taking a holistic approach means keeping an open mind and exploring new ideas. By educating yourself on what is available and trying different things, you can discover what works for you. There is no end to knowledge and what we can discover, no one person or system has all the answers. Knowledge brings power, you no longer feel vulnerable when you discover the power of taking responsibility for yourself.

Maintaining balance is one of the major keys for radiant health. Beneath every problem is an underlying imbalance. Disease cannot take hold in a strong, healthy body. When the immune system is strong and all the organs are functioning properly, the body can successfully fight any infection or virus and also do the repair work of restoration, healing and rejuvenation. However, when the immune system is weak or impaired, it may not have the ability to cope with its every day functions and take on extra work as well. This is why some people get sick easily and others who are exposed to the same bacteria or viruses never get ill. People who get colds and flu every year or who keep taking antibiotics need to strengthen their immune system and replenish their body in the right way.

The combination of a low immune system, high toxicity levels in the body and added pressure from stress or emotional strain cause a decline in health. The root causes of illness are rarely just one factor and for this reason we need to look at as many possible answers through recreating balance in a holistic way and by paying attention to the body, mind, emotions and lifestyle.

Before people get sick, they have usually been overtired or stressed for a period of time, their energy reserves have become depleted and then the immune system breaks down. This does not happen suddenly out of the blue, there are always warning signals, which may have been ignored. The classic response is not now because I don't have the time or the quick fix approach of taking a pill every time there is discomfort in the body. Warning signals that need your attention are feelings of extreme tiredness, not having enough energy, constant irritability or anger, or feeling on overload, which create a pressure cooker effect that could blow up or breakdown at anytime. You cannot exist on zero energy, so unless you do things to nourish and look after yourself, eventually the energy reserves run out.

The body is constantly giving us messages that need to be listened to, discomfort or pain are messages that something needs attention. Continuously taking painkillers, antibiotics, tranquillisers or sleeping pills are desperate quick fixes, which do nothing to resolve the underlying problem. You need to look deeper in order to find the real cause of distress and look for alternative ways of improving your health and promoting healing. Through making some basic changes and becoming more health conscious, you can live a more balanced, higher quality of life.

Creating a New Foundation for Health

The following questionnaire is to help you get an overview of your health and your life. It will give you the opportunity to re-evaluate and understand the foundation upon which radiant health is based. Remember that everything is connected, the physical, mental and emotional and how you think, feel and behave. Read the questionnaire with an open mind but don't make judgements of yourself. Write down or tick the areas that need attention and then list them in order of priority. Throughout the book, you will find many ideas and suggestions, which will help you transform and uplift yourself and develop a new foundation for health.

1. How do you feel when you wake up first thing in the morning?
    Do you wake up feeling fresh and full of energy? Is your mind clear and alert, do you feel eager to start the day? Or do you wake up tired, stiff and needing a cup of tea or coffee to get you going?

2. What are your sleep patterns like?
    How is the quality of your sleep? Do you sleep sound or are you restless and wake up often throughout the night?
    How many hours do you usually sleep?
    Do you get enough sleep or do you have too many late nights?
    What are your dreams like? Do you remember your dreams?

3. How is your energy level?
    Low – never feel as if you have enough
    Okay – could do with more
    Good – generally feel good
    Very good - always full of energy

4. Do you need to take stimulants such as cigarettes, tea or coffee to keep you going throughout the day?

5. How do you feel physically? What sort of imbalances do you have? Any skin or allergy problems, stiffness, pain, discomfort? How is your digestion and elimination?

How is your breathing, is it shallow and restricted or full and expansive?

6. Do you pay attention to your health, both physical and psychological health?
   Do you look for the root cause of problems or do you go for a quick fix?
   Do you follow a preventive health care routine?

7. Do you have a regular fitness programme and pay attention to what you eat and drink? Do you eat when you feel emotional? Do you have cravings?
   Is your weight normal or are you overweight or underweight?

8. Do you take time to relax or meditate or enjoy quiet time when you need it?

9. Do you feel happy and fulfilled with your life?
   If not, do you know why? Are you aware of the changes you need to make to be happier and fulfilled?

10. How do you feel emotionally and psychologically?
    Do your moods fluctuate – a lot or a little?
    Is this at certain times of the month or generally?
    Do you get upset easily? Do you feel depressed, sad, emotionally low or angry – often, occasionally or rarely? What do you do at these times? Do you become self-destructive or have you learnt how to nourish and take care of yourself?

11. Do you suffer from stress – sometimes, often, all the time?
    What are doing about your stress level?

12. Have you created a support programme with different people who can help, guide and support you when you need it? What other support do you need?

13. How clear is your mind, how is your concentration span, how is your short term and long-term memory? How focused are you?

14. Overall how do you feel generally on a physical, mental, psychological and spiritual level? What in you needs attention or healing?

15. Are you using your full potential? Do you express yourself creatively?
Do creative ideas come easily or do you sometimes feel blocked?
Do you feel inspired and enthusiastic about life?
What are you passionate about?

16. Are you following a self-development or spiritual development programme?

17. Do you have good relationships with people both at work and socially?

18. Are you able to express yourself honestly and to ask for what you need?

19. What is the overall picture that you have of yourself?

20. What needs to change in your life?

21. Are you willing to make the necessary changes and to make a commitment to your health, well being and personal growth?

Reprogramming

Before we can make changes in our lives, there has to first be the desire to do so. It won't work if you do it because someone else wants you to; the motivation has to come from within you. If the desire to do something is strong enough then you are bound to achieve it, but if it is weak, it probably won't work. Lethargy and procrastination are obstacles that can get in the way. If you have the tendency to procrastinate, observe it and determine to take another step. Writing down your intentions is helpful and is a way of reminding yourself to keep on track with what you are working towards. In this way, new habits are created. By holding your focus on what you want to achieve, you discover both your strengths and weaknesses. If you find that your motivation is weak or that you keep slipping back into old patterns, find someone to work with who will encourage you to keep going and help you to move through your blocks. Many small steps of positive change can produce an unrecognisable transformation over a period of time.

There is an underlying theme in all natural health programmes, "that if we align ourselves with the laws of nature and come back to what is natural, we will feel happier and be healthier." Coming back to what is natural means coming closer to your real self, your essence and living your truth. Reaching the true self is like peeling back the layers of an onion until we reach the core. Deep inside you know what is right for you but you may go unconscious or no longer trust your intuition because of insecurities, low self-image and fear and from having given your power away to people or things outside of yourself. By developing your listening skills, you will discover a deep intuitive knowingness; it is there in every woman waiting to emerge. By following the whispers of your intuition, you will find it always leads you in the right direction, towards better health, personal growth and more understanding.

In creating a new programme for health and healing, you have to begin with the basics. You need to pay attention to your stress level and bring yourself back to balance by creating a more balanced daily routine, which includes enough rest, relaxation and sleep. You also need to nurture your mind and body with the right food, exercise regularly and supplement your diet with herbs and rejuvenatives. These basics help create a strong foundation for health and prepare you to move deeper into healing, energywork and personal transformation. When you choose to replace dysfunctional habits with more life enhancing ones, nature will support you on every level but first the right conditions have to be created for this to occur.

Stress, a Woman's Greatest Enemy

Stress is a woman's greatest enemy; it breaks down the body's natural defences and accelerates ageing. It is also the root cause of many diseases. Women have a more sensitive nervous system than men and need to take special care not to strain or exhaust themselves. In today's fast moving and demanding world, we have to learn how to cope with stress in a more productive way. Stress has become a household word. Ask almost anyone nowadays if they suffer from stress, and 90% will say yes. Ask what they are doing about it and most people will say nothing and ignore it until a crisis occurs. Stress affects the nervous system, digestion, the reproductive system, the hormones and metabolism. It also depletes our energy level and affects our relationships and performance at work.

What is stress? Stress is the inability to cope with circumstances that appear to be beyond your control or that threaten to overpower you. The outer pressure feels too much and you may feel unable to cope and react to what is going on instead of staying focused and remaining calm and responding to the situation at hand. When you are in a state of reaction, you cannot see clearly, you just want to release the intensity of what you are feeling, it may feel as if you don't have any other choice. Whereas in reality, there is always a choice, you have the choice not to react but instead to remain calm until you become clearer and see what can be done.

Stress is always an inner reaction to an outer situation; it is the result of internal pressure. Stress pushes you into the fear state and this can result in panic attacks, severe stress reactions, exhaustion, chronic fatigue or depression and the breakdown of the nervous and immune system. If you constantly feel that you are on overload and do nothing to release this feeling, long-term this will have debilitating effects on your health. Everyone has to face difficulties and challenges in their lives, but it is how they are handle these situations that makes the difference. Learning to cope with pressure by changing your attitude and detaching and letting go can prevent you from endangering your health. By flowing with the ups and downs of life rather than against it, you can remain more peaceful and take things in your stride.

Women tend to be more sensitive than men and often allow their emotions to overpower them and for this reason statistics show that women suffer more mental disorders and breakdowns. They are also influenced by their hormones and monthly cycles, which can make them moody, anxious or depressed. It is essential during stressful periods to try to maintain one's balance by doing things that nourish you like eating well, getting enough sleep, taking time for yourself, having a massage or a healing session.

Disharmony affects the nervous system, which in turn affects all the other systems of the body. Every experience we have whether positive or negative leaves an imprint in the body; everything is registered including any crisis or trauma. When too many stressful situations occur one on top of each other, a crisis point may be reached and then a breakdown may occur, this could be on a physical, mental or emotional level. You have to learn how to nurture yourself well and not to expect others to do it for you. Do not be afraid to ask for help when you need it, whether it be from friends, a teacher, therapist, healer or a counsellor, do whatever you need to do to put yourself back on track. Don't try to go it alone if you feel really down, help is always there but you may have to reach out and find it. Sometimes what is needed more than anything else is time alone, away from people, to reflect, re-evaluate and come to terms with things. Your health comes first and it is imperative to get the right perspective on this, your health can't wait.

You can learn to deal with stress in a practical way by observing your patterns and limitations. Your feelings are your barometer; they reflect to you what is going on inside of you. You can observe your feelings in a more detached way and without judgement rather than being immersed and lost in them and over reacting. By becoming aware of the first signs of stress and doing something about it, you can prevent a build up, which could have an adverse effect on your physical body.

Whenever you become aware of stress, notice where you hold it in your body. How does it feel, is there tightness or restriction? What happens to your breathing when you feel stressed and does your heart beat faster? How do you react when you get stressed? Do you get panicky or become irritable, snappy, impatient or angry? Watch your stress reactions, come to know them well and then you will be able to master them. As soon as you are aware that you are having a stress reaction, slow down, feel it in your body and take a few minutes to regain your peace of mind. Then breathe slowly and deeply into the area in your body where you are feeling the stress until you feel it dissolve.

What are your automatic responses when you get stressed? Do you reach for a cigarette, coffee, food, crave sweets or something else. Pinpoint your patterns and watch what you do, in this way you can change your automatic responses and transform any destructive or negative behaviour. Find creative and productive ways to discharge your stress on a daily basis; this could be through exercise, relaxation and meditation, cleaning the house, weeding the garden, going for long walks or whatever works for you.

The body has infinite wisdom, it will take every opportunity to respond and heal itself, but if you keep pushing too hard for too long, it will become impossible to retain your natural equilibrium, eventually something will break down. When the nervous system is relaxed and free from stress, then prana, the vital life force flows freely throughout the body and blockages are easily removed. Bodywork and deep relaxation are essential to release tightness and tension from the muscles and to move blocked energy. Treat yourself regularly to some sort of body therapy whether it is massage, reflexology, acupuncture, healing or rebirthing, something that will get the energy moving and help you to release the stress and tension out of the body. (Information on herbs and essences to use for stress, tension and anxiety are given in Chapter 5 - Nature's Gifts)

Rest, Relaxation and Sleep

Most of us live very busy lives and are busy either mentally or physically all day long. In such a fast moving world, rest and relaxation are seen as luxuries, but we are not designed to keep going non-stop like machines, we also need to take time off to recharge our batteries. People who are hyperactive or workaholics find it hard to slow down and even during sleep are still restless and anxious. If you fall into bed exhausted, your body will be tight and the muscles constricted and you will be unable to relax properly during sleep. You may wake in the morning still heavy and drowsy as if you did not get enough sleep and then you may get into an ongoing cycle of restlessness and tiredness, never really feeling rested or refreshed. Many people have forgotten what it means to totally relax the body and get an adequate amount of restful sleep, which are essential for peak mental performance and releasing stress.

Proper relaxation will not only help you to unwind physically and mentally and release the tension from your muscles, it will also take you deeper into yourself. In a state of deep relaxation, you may receive many insights and creative ideas. When I teach Yoga, I always allow time at the end of the class for my students to relax and release. This provides time for integration of the session, to experience the energy flow and to feel the subtle changes that are taking place in the body. In the beginning I see the students have difficulty in relaxing, they can't let go, their minds wander and they are anxious to get up and get on with all the things that they need to do. Then over a period of time, they begin to understand and appreciate the benefits of deep relaxation and really look forward to it.

As the tension from the mind and the body start to release, you are then able to experience what is there in the moment and to shift into a deeper state of consciousness, one of calmness and bliss. Ten to fifteen minutes of deep relaxation before sleeping can change the quality of your sleep and for those who have had chronic sleep problems; it can unwind the tension that has been created over the years. In order for people to experience what it means to deeply relax I have made a CD called "Deep Relaxation, Moving into Stillness."

It is no coincidence that sleep is so often referred to as our beauty sleep, for during sleep the body does its main repair work. Good quality sleep is one of the most important factors in rejuvenation. When the brain and nervous system relax during sleep, then the process of repairing and rebuilding the cells and the tissues takes place. The main detoxification of the body takes place during the hours of 10pm to 2pm, this is the time when the body eliminates toxins, replenishes enzymes and recharges the energy system. By sleeping early as often as possible, you give your body more time to cleanse and regenerate.

People vary on the amount of sleep they need. If you are going through a very active and demanding period in your life or transformational changes, you may find you need more sleep than usual. Most people need between seven to eight hours sleep. You cannot catch up on missed hours of sleep by sleeping late in the morning; it just doesn't work because this interferes with the body's natural rhythms. Over sleeping and sleeping late causes mental sluggishness and depression. Deep fatigue and exhaustion come from many years of not having enough good quality early sleep and not taking the time to rest and relax when you need it. Trying to catch up by sleeping in the day doesn't work either; it makes the brain and metabolism sluggish. It is okay to relax for half an hour in order for the body to unwind and release tension. The exceptions to this are for babies, elderly people or when you are sick and need more sleep in order to recuperate.

When you don't get a good night sleep, your overall performance is affected the next day. You may feel stretched, irritable or impatient and this will affect your communication and relationship with your family or co-workers. What you do in the evening before going to bed also determines the quality of your sleep. If you are a person who tends to be hyperactive or has trouble sleeping, then avoid watching television or working on the computer late at night as this can energize you and make it difficult for you to relax. Try to take at least fifteen minutes of quiet time before sleeping, listen to a tape or soothing music, meditate or read something that won't over stimulate your mind. If we didn't have watches and clocks, we would be more in tune with our body's natural rhythms and automatically sleep when we are tired.

What you eat and drink before sleeping also affects the quality of your sleep. If you eat a heavy meal late at night, your body will have difficulty digesting during the resting phase. If all the energy has to go for digestion and assimilation, then the body cannot do the repair work it is supposed to do during the night. Heavy, late meals in the evening leave you feeling sluggish and unclear the next morning. The earlier and lighter you eat in the evening, the clearer you will feel the next day. People who do a lot of late night entertaining tend to feel tired and dull and need to take stimulants like coffee to keep them going throughout the day.

Avoid taking stimulants in the evening like coffee, black tea or alcohol and if you still have trouble with your sleep, cut them out altogether. Although alcohol seems to relax you, it is classed as a depressant and what it actually does is to produce a drugged state that suppresses the senses and the feelings, it numbs you and in the morning leaves you feeling heavy and the mind dull. If you do have serious sleep problems and are in the habit of taking sleeping pills, try to gradually come off them by finding alternative solutions. Sleeping pills create a zombalistic and depressed state, which does not allow you the benefits of normal, relaxed sleep. There are many combinations of herbs, which can be taken instead.

Massaging your feet with sesame oil and a few drops of lavender oil half an hour before going to sleep and a drop on your temples and the back of the neck can help induce sleep. If you are with a partner, massaging each other's feet for five to ten minutes before sleeping is a wonderful and beneficial way of supporting each other. Children and babies love to have their feet massaged before sleeping too.

You can use essential oils in a burner or place sachets of aromatic herbs that specifically induce sleep under your pillow. It is wonderful to create a regular nightly ritual of burning oils, lighting candles and playing soft music in the bedroom and taking time to unwind before sleep. If your eyes feel tired dab a little rosewater onto cottonwool pads and place them over your eyes, it will help soothe and relax them. Always leave the bedroom window slightly open at night to allow fresh air to circulate in the bedroom; this maintains a fresh supply of oxygen throughout the night. Try to keep the bedroom as clear as possible of clutter so as to create an atmosphere that is relaxing and peaceful. Avoid having electrical equipment in the bedroom, especially a television or computer or electric clock next to the bed; they give off negative vibrations, which are damaging to the nervous system during sleep.

A Balanced Daily Routine

Ayurveda believes that a balanced, daily routine will help restore harmony and is an essential part of any health or healing programme. The balanced daily routine works as a framework that offers certain guidelines and recommendations. We do not have to be rigid in our application for that can also cause tension but to bear in mind that a good routine is beneficial for your well-being. The lack of a daily routine creates instability, which can lead to confusion and depression. If you have a very busy and active lifestyle you can still maintain a certain flexible structure, which encourages you to organize your life around the priorities that are important for you. Then through holding the focus, you draw to you new possibilities and make changes that are in line with your intention.

It is recommended to sleep early and wake early and this will give you clarity of mind and improve your creativity. When you wake up naturally without an alarm clock, which is disturbing to the nervous system, you have time to prepare yourself for the day without having to rush. You can do some Yoga asanas and meditation, have an oil massage and eat a proper breakfast before going off to work. This will make all the difference to how the rest of your day goes. If you get up

23

late and have to rush and there is no time to prepare properly for the day, then this will affect how you feel and behave throughout the rest of your day, it won't be so easy to relax into the day and take what comes in your stride. Taking time in the morning to centre and connect to yourself can make all the difference, even more so when you have important decisions to make.

Likewise how you end the day will affect how you will feel the next day. You want to create a smooth cycle that is supportive of your work and what you want to do. When you are well rested, you are more creative and productive. Ideally it is best to have a light breakfast, a good midday meal and a light supper. This is not always possible for working people although try your best to work around it. The sun is at its highest and most powerful at midday, likewise it is the time when the digestive fire is at its strongest and therefore it is best time to eat the main meal of the day. If you only eat one meal a day, it should be at lunchtime. This is when you body needs more energy during the active phase of the day, whereas in the evening the digestive fire is lower and the body no longer needs so much energy. Eating late in the evening is more of a social activity rather than a necessity for the body.

If you feel tired after eating at lunchtime, this is either because you have eaten too much or the wrong combination of foods, or your digestive power is not strong enough and there may be a problem or weakness in the gastro-intestinal tract. If for some reason due to your work, you cannot eat your main meal at lunchtime, then try to eat as early as possible in the evening and not too heavy. Make sure you eat something at lunchtime, don't skip lunch or live on sandwiches or fast food; lunchtime is the time when your body needs the most nourishment and energy.

The following are some general Ayurvedic guidelines for a balanced daily routine:

- Wake up between 6-7a.m
- Before cleaning your teeth, use a stainless steel tongue scraper to remove the toxins from the tongue.
- Drink a glass of warm water with either one teaspoon of lemon and one teaspoon of honey, or cider vinegar and honey to cleanse and detoxify the body.
- Do a quick exfoliation scrub all over the body with a soft natural bristle brush, followed by 2-3 minutes of body massage with sesame oil. (Longer on weekends or when you have time) Then take your shower or bath.
- Do some morning stretches or Yoga asanas to loosen up the body.
- Meditate to prepare you for the day.
- Take a light breakfast
- Eat your main meal at lunchtime. Even if time is short, be quiet and relaxed whilst eating and eat slowly.
- In the evening, before eating do some exercise or Yoga asanas or go for a walk after dinner.
- Meditate before dinner or before going to sleep.
- Eat lightly in the evening and as early as possible and do not eat any late night snacks.
- Drink a herbal tea if desired half an hour before sleeping to help you relax.
- Sleep as often as possible by 10-10.30p.m (Remember sleep is the great rejuvenator.)

Exercise

Exercise is an important part of any health regime. Ideally one should do some sort of exercise every day especially if you have a job that requires you to sit a lot during the day. Some people like to go to the gym; others prefer to bicycle, jog or walk or to play a sport. There is such a variety to choose from. Whatever you decide to do, try to maintain a regular routine. Regularity is the key and it takes discipline to keep going but regular exercise will make a big difference long term to how you feel. If you lack discipline, arrange to go with a friend so that you can motivate each other. At times when you don't really feel like it, do less but still continue, take it gently or change to another form of exercise that might suit you better. People who exercise regularly feel more energized and more enthusiastic. Once you experience how much better you feel when you exercise regularly, you will never want to give it up.

I emphasize an exercise routine that works for you. All exercise routines should begin gently and gradually build up. If you haven't been exercising regularly then start with something easy like a brisk daily walk or a few Yoga stretches or dancing to your favourite music. Straining or leaving the gym feeling worn out is counter productive and is not going to encourage you to keep going. Aerobic classes may be great for the young or super fit but can be a strain for the average woman who has a lot of responsibilities. Over exercising can make you feel weak and tired and is not advisable. Listen to your body and respect its present limitations and gradually build up your strength and vitality. You need to create an exercise routine that is going to make you feel good, move your energy, increase your circulation, strengthen your muscles and relieve tension. Exercise oxygenates the brain and improves memory and alertness and transforms depression. A lack of exercise results in inflexibility, restricted energy flow and a build up of toxicity and acidity, which causes pain in the muscles and joints and premature ageing.

Different body types need different types of exercise. A strong, heavy body type with a good constitution will need to do more working out and can jog and sweat without feeling exhausted, whereas a lightweight, slim body type will tire more easily and is in need of a gentler form of exercise. The type of exercise you choose can vary, you don't always have to do the same thing everyday. Exercise should be something you look forward to and enjoy and this will also depend on your lifestyle and how much time you have available. If it is an effort to get to the gym or a class everyday, plan to go once or twice a week and also workout for 15-30 minutes every day at home in between. My personal choice of exercise is Yoga, this has been an important part of my life for many years and one of the wonders of Yoga is that you can practise it until any age. (More on Yoga in Chapter 4 - Rejuvenation).

Nowadays there is a tendency towards a more sedentary lifestyle and when we feel tired we may be reluctant to exercise but if you push yourself gently through the resistance, afterwards you will see that you feel so much better. If you want to work towards a high level of health and fitness, you should try to exercise at least twenty minutes to half an hour every day. I advise my clients to do some simple Yoga standing and stretching exercises first thing in the morning to get the energy moving and to prepare them for the day and some sitting and lying Yoga asanas in the evening. Walking is also a wonderful way of relieving stress and tension. If you walk in the evening, it helps you to unwind from the day and improves the quality of your sleep. On weekends try to get out and walk for longer periods of time, preferably in nature if you can.

As well as stretching, you also need some sort of regular aerobic exercise to get the heart pumping efficiently and to improve your lung capacity. Aerobic exercise (here I don't mean the aerobic exercises, which are taught in many gyms) also helps build up stamina and increases blood and lymph circulation, this has a cleansing effect and increases the calcium content of the bones. You can choose from walking, dancing, swimming, cycling or a sport. A good investment is to buy a mini trampoline, also known as a rebounder. You can jump or dance on it to your favourite music, it is great fun, very enlivening and the children will love it too and it is an easy way to get a regular cardiovascular workout. Jumping or dancing on the trampoline for 10-15 minutes every day, is the equivalent of an aerobic workout and a wonderful stress releaser.

Remember to drink enough water before and after exercising, this helps flush out the toxins that have been released whilst exercising.

Do not eat for at least three hours before exercising, if you eat a heavy meal, you may need to allow longer.

Whilst you exercise, keep your attention on your body and be aware of your breath. If your breathing becomes too fast, this means you are straining and need to slow down. Always listen carefully to your body whilst exercising, never strain or push beyond your comfortable capacity, instead allow your body to build up strength and stamina by gradually increasing your fitness level.

2 - CONSCIOUS EATING

Ayurveda considers food to be powerful medicine. Hippocrates, the father of modern medicine said, "Let food be your medicine." Eating the right food and the right amount of food, as well as fasting occasionally promotes regeneration and nourishes and rebuilds the body. If we see food as medicine rather than something just to fill us up or to satisfy the emotions and the senses, we will change our attitude towards food.

The whole subject of food and what we eat has become a highly emotional subject. Many emotional disorders manifest as eating disorders, including weight problems, obesity, food intolerances, allergies, addictions and anorexia and bulimia, which are on the increase especially amongst young women. There are underlying stress related problems, which make people turn to food as a substitute for other things. We have to identify what the underlying feelings are and not keep pushing down those feelings with food, which does nothing to alleviate the real problem.

Addictions to any substance whether food, including sugar, coffee, cigarettes, alcohol or drugs or overeating are all related to one's emotional state and feelings. There may be feelings of dissatisfaction, inadequacy, lack of fulfilment or not feeling loved. This is the reason why so many people procrastinate and put things off, they are always going to start a new diet, new exercise programme etc When they try to change their diet all sorts of resistance and reactions come up; it brings up the underlying emotional patterns. Changes need to be made gradually, if necessary get professional support whilst making these changes. Don't be hard on yourself or criticize yourself, just try to become more conscious of what you are doing and why you do it and endeavour to gradually change the patterns and habits. Emotional eating is a cry for another kind of nourishment. This chapter deals mainly with nourishing your physical body, which also affects how you feel and think. In the following chapters you will find many other ways to nourish yourself both emotionally and spiritually.

A vast number of people suffer from nutritional deficiencies. They are literally starved of high quality, pure energy giving food and this is not because it is not available but because there is a lot of misinformation around the subject of food and eating. It has become fashionable in some countries to take large doses of chemically produced vitamins, which are hard for the body to digest. Taking handfuls of vitamins every day cannot supplement eating properly or fulfil the body's desire for real sustenance and nourishment.

Everything you ingest has an affect on your physical body, your energy level, your mind and the way you feel. Certain foods increase your energy level and nourish and supply the fuel for the proper functioning of the body and the production of new, healthy cells, whilst others dull or block the body and offer no real sustenance. By feeding the cells of the body with high quality, high-energy content foods you can change the whole cellular structure of the body including the brain. In this way, you can recreate the basic building blocks of the body. If you ingest poor quality food, your health will be poor. When the cells of the body are deprived of proper nutrition and life force energy, they begin to deteriorate and imbalances occur which lead to mutations, disease and premature ageing. Poor diet is a major factor in most diseases including heart disease, cancer and tumours.

If you overeat or overindulge, neglect or abuse your body, the results will become apparent in your health and affect your mind including memory and concentration span. If your mind is dull or you suffer from constant fatigue, look at your eating habits to find some of the answers. Conscious eating and including other life enhancing habits can change how you feel and improve your energy level. When you have more energy, you naturally feel better.

To become free from cravings and emotional addictions and to develop discrimination as to what is really good for you, you have to become more health and body conscious. Before eating anything get into the habit of asking yourself is this nourishing for my body and mind? Does it contain life force energy? Is this really good for me or am I eating or drinking it to satisfy my emotions or senses. Then make the choice whether you still want to eat or drink it. This is conscious eating.

Optimum Nutrition

Optimum nutrition is a term used for giving the best quality food to your body. It means eating for health in order to feed and nourish the cells of the body in the best possible way, giving them the optimum nutrition that they require. When we adopt this way of looking at food, it changes our whole perspective towards eating. When you go shopping, buy with the intention of giving your body the best possible quality food; choose the freshest food you can find and preferably organic. Think in terms of promoting health, vitality and rejuvenation. We need to eat food that is full of life force energy.

There are different types of foods known as biogenic and bioacidic. Biogenic foods are life generating; they are alive and full of life force energy and. have cell renewing capabilities and restore proper hormone and enzyme balance. Bioacidic foods have no life force and upset the chemical balance of the body and foster degeneration.

Ayurveda classifies foods into three categories, sattvic, tamasic and rajasic. Sattvic food is that which is soothing and nourishing for the mind and body. It creates stability, rejuvenates and prolongs long life. It is also food that has a soothing effect upon the body and is easily digestible. Some examples of sattvic foods are fresh spring water, ghee, fresh fruit and freshly made fruit juices, raw foods, basmati rice, yellow mung beans, freshly cooked vegetables, wheat, oats, sesame oil, almonds, honey, dates and coconut.

Tamasic food is what is considered to be dead food, it has no nutritional content and it contains no life force energy, no vitamins or minerals. Tamasic food has a dull influence on the mind and the body and makes you feel lethargic. Examples of tamasic foods are frozen, tinned and preserved foods, leftovers and old food, junk food, microwaved food and foods containing preservatives, chemicals or colourings or any foods which could be classed as unnatural.

Rajasic food irritates the body and has a debilitating effect on the mind and nervous system. Examples of rajasic foods are those which are too hot, too spicy, too salty, chilies, garlic, onions, tomatoes, aubergines, meat, alcohol, black tea, coffee, cigarettes, sugary foods, soft drinks, crisps and fermented foods such as cheese and vinegar.

As you include more sattvic foods in your diet, you will notice a difference in your energy level. Sattvic foods contain prana, the universal life force energy and this has a direct affect on the nervous system and the energy system.

Certain foods also have special medicinal or antibiotic properties as well as having a nourishing and healing affect. These foods are known as superfoods and you should include as many of these regularly in your diet.

Superfoods

In essence all raw, fresh foods, preferably organic are rejuvenating foods since they contain many nutrients including enzymes, which are the life force of food.

It is essential to drink at least one litre of fresh, spring water every day. Don't drink tap water, which may be polluted and full of chemicals. Most people are dehydrated and this causes many unexplained problems and pain in the body. You can energize your water by putting it in a glass jar or container with a clean quartz crystal in it and leaving it in the sun for about ten to fifteen minutes, this will purify the water. If you are unable to obtain bottled water, then boil the water for about ten minutes to make sure that it is safe to drink.

Eat plenty of fresh fruit, and drink fresh fruit juices and fresh vegetable juices every day (fresh as in homemade and freshly juiced, packaged juices are usually heated to preserve them, this creates acidity.) Fresh juices contain a high percentage of life force energy. Fresh, natural juice will rehydrate your body. Fruit is an excellent cleanser and helps eliminate impurities from the body. It is said that fresh fruit in the morning is like gold for the body. Select fruits that are sweet and ripe not sour and preferably in season.

Fruit juices and all fruits should be eaten separately from other foods. The exception to this is apples; they can be mixed with other foods. Never eat fruit after a meal as this causes acidity. Citrus fruits can change an acidic condition of the body to alkaline. Choose from oranges, lemons, grapefruit, apples, grapes and watermelon juice. If oranges are sour, they can cause acidity, drink orange juice in moderation as it is known to cause headaches and allergic reactions in some people. Carrot juice is one of the most nourishing juices and is good to drink everyday. It can be mixed with apple and celery and other green foods. You can also mix carrot juice with a little beetroot and celery juice and/or parsley and coriander.

It is healthy to drink one fruit juice daily and one green or mixed juice daily. To make a green juice, combine any of the following, celery, spinach, parsley, coriander, spinach, cabbage, any green leafy vegetables and cucumbers. Green juices are energy drinks; they detoxify and alkalise the blood, nourish the nerves, and are a tonic for the brain and immune system. They are chlorophyll rich and are an excellent source of vitamins, minerals, protein and enzymes. You can dilute the juice by adding water or fresh apple to sweeten.

Grapes and apples are powerful intestinal cleansers, apples are cleansing for the gall bladder and lower cholesterol. They are also good for the lungs and prevent respiratory problems. They contain pectin, which helps eliminate toxic metals. There is a phytochemical in apples, which has an inhibitory effect on cancer and tumour formation, so eat at least one apple every day. Watermelon is a diuretic, it flushes toxins from the kidneys and neutralizes acids, carrots contains beta carotene which is recognized as a cancer fighting nutrient, cucumbers stimulate the kidneys, parsley is a blood purifier and diuretic and beetroot stimulates the liver and purifies the blood. Cranberry juice is helpful for urinary tract infections, including cystitis. Melon does not mix well with other fruits or foods; eat it at the beginning of the meal and avoid eating it with cheese or meat, as is the custom in some countries, this causes gastric problems.

Avocado has been called the king of the fruit kingdom. It is a complete food, containing protein and vitamin A, B, C and E, and is rich in potassium.

Aloe Vera juice should be taken on a daily basis. It detoxifies the blood and the lymph system and aids and heals stomach and digestive tract problems including acidity. It can be taken ongoing as a digestive aid and tonic. If you don't like the taste, you can add it to fresh juice.

Chlorella is a green superfood. It is a micro-algae, which is found in lakes. It contains the highest level of chlorophyll amongst all known foods and also contains physiologically activating substances. It has a very high level of protein, so is excellent for vegetarians, it also contains many vitamins including Vitamin B12, minerals and amino acids. Spirolina and bluegreen algae are two other well-known greenfoods.

Beehive products including pollen rich honey, propolis and royal jelly are considered to be superfoods. (See Chapter 4 - Rejuvenation) It is recommended to add honey to all natural remedies to increase their potency.

Ghee is clarified butter. Through a simple process of heating butter, the milk solids are removed. Ghee is considered in Ayurveda to be a rasayana, (health promoting) and to be one of the most nourishing and sattvic foods (see more on ghee in Chapter 4 -

Rejuvenation) and a recipe on how to make ghee at the end of this chapter.

Sprouted seeds are full of nutrients, enzymes, and life force energy. Sprouted alfalfa, soya beans, sunflower and pumpkin seeds are an excellent source of calcium, protein and B vitamins. They can easily be grown in containers or trays. Soak them first overnight to encourage the germination process and then put them into a container and rinse with fresh water several times a day. Alfalfa has been described as a miracle legume and can be eaten daily; it helps restore the acid/alkaline balance. It is interesting that such a delicate little plant contains so many vitamins, minerals and enzymes.

Kelp is nutritious seaweed, it is the best source of iodine other than fish or sea vegetables and highly recommended for vegetarians. It is rich in minerals including calcium, magnesium, potassium, phosphorus, iron, and carotene. It is a nutritive tonic, which balances the metabolism and is especially beneficial for the thyroid. It is also an antioxidant.

There are four main types of sea vegetables or seaweeds; they are Hijiki, which is rich in potassium, Dulse, which is rich in iron and Wakame and Kombu. Try to either include one of these in your diet if you don't eat fish or take kelp.

Lecithin, has been called brain food, it feeds the brain tissues. It lowers cholesterol and aids in the digestion of fat and helps in weight loss, it also protects the gall bladder. It is found in soya beans and soya milk. Lecithin granules can be sprinkled on food.

Olive oil has been called the king of the oils; it is the richest source of vitamin E, which is essential for rejuvenation. It is an antioxidant and destroys free radicals. It is good for the gall bladder and the prevention of stones and lowers cholesterol. Use it in salads and in cooking; take 1 tablespoon of olive oil a day. It is very good for the skin. Buy cold pressed, high-grade virgin olive oil.

Fresh coriander is an antioxidant, full of vitamins, minerals and enzymes and is unique in its ability to flush heavy metals out of the body. It helps excrete mercury (from amalgam fillings), lead and aluminium. Add coriander to green juices, salads and rice dishes.

Take a daily dose of essential fatty acids, 1 teaspoon each of sesame, sunflower and pumpkin seeds. Grind a few tablespoons of each, mix them well and store in the fridge. The seeds are a good source of protein and minerals including zinc and vitamin E. They are also good for the reproductive organs. Essential fatty acids are also found in evening primrose oil, starflower oil and borage oil, there are nutritional supplements, which contain all three oils.

Linseeds also known as Flaxseeds are rich in Omega 3 fatty acids, B vitamins, potassium, magnesium, zinc and protein. These little seeds have an amazing amount of benefits, especially for the immune system, as they are anti-viral, antibacterial and antifungal. They are helpful in inflammation, pain and swelling in the joints and good for strong bones, teeth, nails, pressure in the eyes, water retention, blood clotting, colon problems, constipation and as a protection for the heart by keeping the arteries clean of cholesterol. Grind and sprinkle 1-2 teaspoons a day on food.

Almonds are known as the king of the nuts. They have a very high protein value and contain many vital minerals and B vitamins. Take 8-10 skinned almonds a day.

Lentils contain anti cancer compounds called inhibitors. Mung dhal (found in Indian shops and some health food shops) is considered to be the most nutritious and the easiest bean to digest. They can be eaten every day and added to soups, rice and vegetable dishes.

Black molasses is a natural wonder beverage; it is very rich in calcium, iron, phosphorus, and potassium. It is a rich source of vitamin B, especially high in B6.

It feeds the brain cells and the nervous system and is helpful for arthritis, tumours, skin problems, detoxification and constipation. Take 1 tsp a day or more if needed in warm water before meals.

Apple cider vinegar has an alkalising effect. It dissolves calcium deposits and kidney stones, aids virus infections, lowers high blood pressure, fights infections, relieves arthritis and rheumatism, flushes the gall bladder and is helpful in osteoporosis because it feeds the bones. It contains 93 different components and is very rich in minerals. Take 1-2 tsp apple cider vinegar with 1 tsp of honey first thing in the morning, in warm water for a cleansing effect and as a general tonic. You can also make herbal apple cider vinegar by adding 1 cup of herbs to 2 cups of apple cider vinegar. Select from a mixture of bay leaves, dill, lemon balm, basil, parsley, rosemary, thyme and coriander. (Ordinary vinegar is very acidic and should be avoided.)

Dried fruits such as dates, figs, prunes, raisins and apricots are concentrated sources of nutrients and energy. They are rich sources of iron, potassium and calcium. Bedouin Arabs travel across the desert for days eating only dates and figs. Soak a combination of dried fruits in water over night and eat them for breakfast the next morning, also drink the juice. (Soaking makes them easily digestible.) Raisins in particular have medicinal value; they are good for the brain and for the respiratory system and the bowels. Include 2 tablespoons with your food every day but avoid golden coloured raisins, which have been treated.

Oats have a high content of vitamin B, they are a wonderful balancing and grounding food and they increase stamina. Oats are especially good for women as they have a restorative effect on the nervous system. They are good to eat when you need sustenance. Because of their balancing effect, they are helpful when having withdrawal effects from giving up cigarettes, alcohol or drugs. They also contain a substance that lowers cholesterol.

Broccoli is considered a super green food and has remarkable anti-aging properties. It is very high in chlorophyll and good for the reproductive tissue.

It is important to include some fibre in your diet; it keeps the bowels regular and protects the colon by removing cancer causing particles from the body. It helps regulate blood sugar levels, reduces cholesterol and lowers blood pressure. Good sources of fibre are all unrefined carbohydrates, fruit, vegetables, whole grains, oatmeal, and cereals.

Fresh yoghurt contains acidophilus, which helps prevent putrefaction in the intestines and increases the beneficial bacteria. Yogurt helps build immunity when eaten every day. It is not mucus forming like milk. Lassi is a drink made from natural yoghurt and can be taken with or before meals as a digestive aid. It is made from half yoghurt and half water and can be sweetened with rosewater, carob juice, cinnamon or nutmeg.

Noni is a medicinal, healing fruit found in tropical areas such as Polynesia and Hawaii. It is said to have curative qualities that enhance the body's healing abilities. It helps bring about homeostasis through a balancing effect, which can normalize blood pressure (whether high or low) and sugar levels and is said to relieve many ailments including inhibiting the growth of tumours and malignant cells. (See more on Noni in Chapter 4 - Rejuvenation).

Other Medicinal Foods

Carob juice or carob powder contains three times as much calcium as milk. Carob juice makes a healthy drink and can be added to cereals or yoghurt.

Ginger root is a major medicinal food in China; it aids digestion by increasing the digestive fire. It is an antioxidant that kills bacteria and fungi, reduces cholesterol and prevents blood clots. It clears ama, a sticky substance that forms in the channels of the body. It can be grated and added to salads or used in cooking. It can also be drunk daily as a tea to improve digestion, add a few slices of fresh ginger root to a cup of boiled water and allow it to cool. Drink the ginger tea before meals or eat a couple of slices of fresh ginger with your food.

Garlic is a natural antibiotic; it helps with infections and kills parasites, viruses and fungi. It is good for the heart and can be taken for both high and low blood pressure, for high cholesterol, and blood clotting. It is better for the heart than any manmade drug. Its medicinal uses were mentioned in the earliest Vedic literature, it was even used for amoebic dysentery. Kyolic garlic, which is preserved in a special way is taken in tablet form and has the advantage that it does not smell. However, it should be mentioned that although garlic can be taken as a medicine for short periods of time and for a specific purpose, it is not recommended to take it on going, both garlic and onions have a rajasic, irritating effect on the mind and nervous system.

Onion juice helps clear bacterial infections especially in the throat. Make onion tea by boiling 3-4 cut onions in approximately a litre of water, bring to the boil and simmer for 10 minutes, allow to cool and strain, drink throughout the day. Take onion tea for three consecutive days or until the infection clears.

Kefir is a substance similar to yoghurt, which aids in digestive problems and helps recreate natural bacterial balance in the gut. It is helpful where candida is present in the body.

Soya beans, chickpeas, bean sprouts, asparagus, tomatoes, potatoes and oats have a natural antibiotic effect and help fight infections, they also protect against parasites. Carrots, broccoli, spinach, winter squash, turnips, cabbage and brussel sprouts contain anticancer substances and should be eaten regularly. Parsley has a cleansing effect by increasing circulation. Bananas are good when there is diarrhoea or loose stools, but they should be avoided if there is a tendency towards constipation or asthma. Cabbage juice is helpful for acidity and ulcers. Shred the cabbage, boil it and then drink the water.

Fennel is a digestive aid and dispels mucus; it can also help with morning sickness. Parsnips, sweet potatoes, yams and squash are root vegetables that strengthen the internal organs and give the body energy. Grapefruit seed is helpful for yeast infection, fungus, viruses, parasites, salmonella and traveller's diarrhoea. Soaked, dried apricots relieve constipation and clean the intestinal wall. Radishes and asparagus help purify the blood and urine. Replace regular black tea with green tea, which is rich in antioxidants and protects against cancer.

It is very healthy to cook with spices, which have medicinal and therapeutic properties. You can sauté spices in ghee and then add the vegetables or rice or pour the ghee and spices over the vegetables and rice afterwards. Spices help the body assimilate nutrients from the food. Adding spices to the cooking, especially cumin, black pepper and fresh ginger reduce the gassy effect or bloatedness that some people experience especially when eating beans. Ayurveda has specially prepared spice mixtures for each particular body type that are suitable for particular imbalances. The following are some of the most popular spices and their therapeutic effects.

If there is one spice you should use regularly, it is turmeric, which is considered to be an all round wonder spice. Turmeric has anti cancer properties, (it protects the DNA of the cell), it is anti inflammatory, anti-allergic, antifungal and a natural antibiotic. It stimulates digestion, detoxifies the liver, boosts the immune system and balances cholesterol levels.

To increase heat in the body add warming spices such as ginger, cinnamon, nutmeg or black pepper. To decrease heat in the body add cumin, liquorice or fennel. Cinnamon is a warming, stimulating spice, which is helpful for circulation and digestive problems, but it should not be taken during pregnancy. Nutmeg is another warming spice that is good for digestive problems and is considered to be an aphrodisiac for increasing sexual libido. It must only be taken in very small amounts. Black pepper is another warming spice, known for its cleansing and antioxidant properties. It helps the free flow of oxygen to the brain, enhances digestion and stimulates the appetite.

Clove has antiseptic, antibacterial and antispasmodic properties and can help eliminate parasites. It is helpful in mouth, gum and throat infections. Saffron is a balancing spice and helps flush toxins out of the body. Ginger helps clear bad breath by improving digestion and stimulating the digestive fire. Liquorice balances the liver and is a cooling spice, which is ideal for menopausal women. Cumin is another cooling spice, which aids digestion and flushes out toxins. Fennel is also a cooling spice that is good for digestion. In India it is the custom to eat a few fennel seeds after every meal to aid digestion. Coriander helps cellular detoxification and eliminates heavy metals from the body.

Vitamins and Minerals

If you eat a diet that is high in vitamins and minerals and eat a variety of foods including enough of the recommended superfoods and add natural food supplements, this should cover your daily vitamin and mineral requirements. The exception to this is if you have been diagnosed with a specific deficiency or disease and therefore need more of a particular vitamin or mineral. In most cases, this can still be corrected through dietary changes by adding natural food supplements and rasayanas (tonic herbs) to your daily diet. The overuse of insecticides and modern farming methods have resulted in poor quality soil which lacks an abundance of minerals and vital trace elements, but by including specific superfoods such as aloe vera juice, chlorella or other algae, kelp, bee hive products and apple cider vinegar and coral calcium, we can boost our mineral requirements to the optimum level. Complex chemical vitamin and mineral supplements are difficult for the body to digest and assimilate and do not enliven and nourish the cellular level of the body as do prana rich, living foods. Chemicals cannot replace natural life force energy.

Aloe vera juice is mainly known for its cleansing and healing properties but it is also very rich in nutritional elements. It contains 75 different nutrients, vitamins, minerals, antioxidants, 20 amino acids (the building blocks of the body) and enzymes. It is one of the few plant sources containing B12, which is essential for vegetarians. It is rare for one plant to contain so many minerals; it is rich in magnesium, manganese, zinc, copper, chromium, calcium, sodium, potassium and iron. The quality of aloe vera juice varies a lot, some are watery and contain almost no sap, so make sure to buy the best you can find.

The following is a list of vitamins and minerals and the main vegetarian sources they can be found in:

Vitamin A is necessary for a strong immune system and helps fight cancer. The best sources are carrots (drink carrot juice daily), dandelion tea, green leafy vegetables, spinach, cabbage, parsley, tomatoes, dried apricots, broccoli, sweet potato and pumpkin.

A lack of vitamin B causes mental sluggishness, poor memory and moodiness. The best sources of Vitamin B are found in sunflower seeds, almonds, wheatgerm, soybeans and soya products, broccoli, lentils, yoghurt, avocados and black molasses. Vitamin B6 is found in wheat, wheatgerm, oats, walnuts, soya products, avocados, raisins and bee pollen. B12 is found in Aloe vera juice and chlorella.

Vitamin C is vital for the immune system and helps increase the natural production of interferon, the body's own defence chemical. Red pepper has the highest content of vitamin C. Other good sources are parsley, dandelion, nettles, green leafy vegetables, broccoli, citrus fruits, apples, melon, berries, potatoes and sweet potatoes.

Vitamin D we take from the sun. The sun is a source of energy for both the body and the mind. Vitamin D is necessary for calcium absorption and healthy bones. You need exposure to the sun every day. People who do not get enough sunlight may suffer from depression. Vitamin D is also found in fish oils and cereals.

Vitamin E improves circulation to the brain, boosts the immune system and helps protect against infection. It prevents blood clotting and neutralizes cancer-causing chemicals. The best sources are vegetable oils, the best being olive oil and wheatgerm oil, nuts, seeds especially linseeds (flaxseeds), olives, wheatgerm, almonds and avocados, grains, green leafy vegetables and green drinks.

The best source of iron is black molasses, iron is also found in kelp, soya products, pumpkin, sunflower and pumpkin seeds, sea vegetables, wheat products including wheatgerm, green leafy vegetables, broccoli, courgettes, avocados, beets, alfalfa, dandelion, parsley, prunes, wholegrain bread, cereals, oats, almonds, lentils, raisins, Nettle, lapacho and sideritis tea, which is a herb that is unique to the Mediterranean and has a high iron content.

Magnesium is important for skeletal development, for the bones and the tissues, it is found in soya products, dried apricots, bananas, kelp, green vegetables, dandelion, dates, avocados, raisins, seeds, nuts, whole grain cereals, seafood, pulses, apples, potatoes and broccoli.

Potassium is an essential key mineral necessary for the metabolic process and to keep the tissues soft and pliable, it also helps alkalise the body, the main sources are dried apricots, figs, raisins, dates, prunes, sea vegetables, root vegetables, brazil nuts, walnuts, spinach, parsley, avocados, parsnips, squash, honey and molasses.

Zinc is important for the reproductive system, for regeneration and healing, it is found in pulses, wheatgerm, oats, almonds, linseeds, sunflower and pumpkin seeds and bee pollen.

Selenium, which has been called the anti-ageing mineral, is an important antioxidant and trace element, which preserves the skin's elasticity. It is found in brazil nuts, cabbage, rice and noni juice. Smoking depletes selenium and other minerals.

Copper is an essential mineral that purifies the digestive system, reduces acidity and improves assimilation. Wear a copper bracelet or fill a copper cup with water overnight, during the night the cup will absorb the copper and first thing in the morning drink the water.

Boron helps prevent the loss of calcium, phosphorus and magnesium, it is found in dried apricots, alfalfa, cabbage, lettuce, peas, apples, dates, prunes, raisins and almonds.

Protein and Calcium

Protein is necessary to repair and maintain the cells, tissues, bones and muscles. The body produces certain enzymes and hormones, which create protein. Most people eat too much protein and not the right kind of protein. Excess protein from animal products contributes to heart disease, arthritis, osteoporosis and strokes. Milk and milk products are hard to metabolise and can create excess mucus in the respiratory system. Milk is considered to be one of the highest allergy foods and it contains a lot of hormones, which can imbalance the reproductive system. Avoid drinking ice cold milk, which interferes with digestion or drinking milk with meals, as it does not combine well with other foods. If you drink milk, it is best to boil it first and then add spices to makes it more digestible. Avoid all dairy products if you have respiratory problems especially asthma. Fresh yoghurt contains certain bacteria that help the digestive system. Do not eat yoghurt that is more than a day old as it become sour and looses its value. Hard cheeses create uric acid, which weakens the bones and causes arthritis and osteoporosis.

Vegetable protein is important for the efficient functioning of the pituitary gland. It is known that a vegetarian diet can prevent 97% of coronary heart disease. Protein from vegetable sources is easier to digest and does not block the circulatory channels. The best sources of vegetable protein are from lentils, mung dhal, chickpeas, potatoes, rice and other grains, nuts and seeds. Mung dhal and basmati rice form a complete protein. It is recommended to eat some type of beans and rice at least twice a week.

Soya products and soya milk have been recommended as ideal sources of protein instead of dairy products. There are some questions being raised recently and conflicting information about soya milk, which is made from uncooked soya beans and whether it is actually good for us or not, we will no doubt be hearing more about this, as information becomes available. Choose soya products that have not been genetically engineered and consume them in only small amounts. Soya milk should not be given to children because of the hormonal type substance that it contains or taken by breast feeding mothers. Soya also contains genostein, which is said to protect against cancer. Tofu is one of the best soya products to eat.

Calcium is needed for healthy bones, teeth, blood and the nervous system and the best vegetarian sources are yoghurt, sea vegetables, kelp, almonds, (eat 10 a day) sunflower seeds, sesame seeds, walnuts, almonds, prunes, dried figs, black molasses, tofu, carob, oats, and plenty of green vegetables. Citrus fruits also contain calcium and phosphorus and are found in lemons, limes, grapefruit, oranges and mandarins. Cottage cheese and anari can be eaten in small amounts. Excessive amounts of calcium from eating too much animal protein causes kidney stones in adults. Coral calcium, also known as alkamine, is one of the best natural sources of calcium and also contains magnesium and many other minerals. (See the osteoporosis section in chapter 6).

Dietary Principles of Balanced Nutrition

By following the dietary principles of balanced nutrition, you can aid the digestive and assimilation processes and prevent dietary imbalances, which can lead to discomfort or ill health.

1. Keep meals simple and don't eat too many different foods at any one meal. People often feel tired or uncomfortable after dinner parties or buffet dinners because of eating too many different foods at a time, which is confusing for the body. Choose foods, which are light and easy for the body to digest.

2. Don't overeat, it blocks the body and creates excess waste, which becomes excess weight and is hard to lose. When eating, the stomach should only be filled to the capacity of two thirds full; the one third should be left for the digestive juices to work. Resist having second helpings of food and instead leave the table feeling satisfied but not completely full. Try to be aware of how much food your body really needs and learn to recognize what is emotional eating or greediness. Over indulging causes weight gain, high acidity levels and can damage the DNA, thereby increasing the possibility of mutations and cancer.

3. For the food to be well digested and assimilated, agni, the digestive fire needs to be strong and active. If agni is low, the digestive process will be impaired and slow and foods will not be properly digested. Overeating puts out the digestive fire and prevents proper assimilation and then you have cravings for more food because the cells have not received enough nutrients. If you feel tired after eating, you have either eaten too much or your digestive fire is low. Over eating also causes mental dullness.

4. The digestive fire is the strongest at lunchtime, when the sun is at its highest. It is therefore advisable to eat the main meal of the day at lunchtime; this is also when the body needs the most energy. To stimulate the digestive fire, eat fresh ginger with your food or add it to cooking or drink ginger tea (hot water with a few slices of fresh ginger) throughout the day.

5. Eat lightly in the evening and as early as possible. The body does not need so much energy in the evening when it is slowing down and preparing for rest and rejuvenation. Late, heavy meals make you feel tired and sluggish the next morning and accumulate weight. If you want to lose weight, cut out the evening meal or eat very little in the evening.

6. Avoid eating in between meals, the exception to this is fruit or fruit juices, but wait until the food has been digested. Eating in

between meals (other than fruit) weakens the digestive power and creates a build up of toxins, excess weight and cellulite. You need at least three to four hours to digest a main meal and one to two hours to digest snacks (longer for meat). If you eat a main meal and then eat a snack before the meal is digested, then you are mixing undigested food with partially digested food and neither will be properly digested. If you keep snacking throughout the day, the body will be confused and the digestive juices will keep working and this will result in excess acidity and create a toxic environment.

7. If you want to eat more food or to snack after having eaten, recognize that this is not hunger but an emotional craving and try to resist eating more. To cut the craving drink lots of hot water and ginger and when it has cooled, add a little honey, this can also satisfy sweet cravings.

8. Avoid drinking with food except for a little water, this is a social habit and not a healthy one, it dilutes the digestive juices. Don't drink straight after a meal, wait for at least an hour.

9. At different times of year and depending on our body type and the climate we live in, we need different types of food. In summer, we need more cooling foods; we are naturally drawn more towards more cleansing and lighter foods, especially raw foods, salads, fresh fruits and juices. In winter, we need more nourishing and heavier, warm foods, soups, cooked vegetables, grains and beans. Warm foods increase metabolism and are easier to digest. If your digestive power is low or weak, it is better to eat warm, cooked foods until your agni increases. If you are a person who tends to feel the cold and has a vata constitution, you will feel better eating warming foods and hot drinks. If you have a lot of heat in your body and always feel warm, this indicates a strong pitta (fire) element, you will prefer cooling foods and drinks. (Avoid ice cold drinks or cold food straight from the fridge, which put out the digestive fire). Listen to your body and make the necessary adjustments to your diet at different times of the year.

10. In the summer months, it is beneficial to drink only fresh fruit juices and to eat only fruit until lunchtime. Fruit juices and fruit are nourishing, energizing and cleansing. It is not so suitable however during the winter months or if you live in a cold climate. You can still start your day with a fresh fruit juice, wait fifteen minutes and then eat your breakfast or drink your juice or eat fruit midmorning. Remember not to mix fruit with other foods and to eat it before a meal not afterwards as this creates fermentation and acidity, which draws calcium out of the bones.

11. There are a lot of different opinions on whether to eat raw food or cooked food. Raw food is full of live enzymes and has a cleansing effect but if you suddenly eat lots of raw food, you may develop toxic reactions or allergies may be activated, you have to introduce it slowly. If the digestive fire is not strong enough or assimilation is slow, too much raw food can cause bloating or discomfort in the intestines, especially if there are too many toxins in the digestive tract. Cooked food is easier to digest. It is good to include some raw food every day in your diet and to eat more during the summer months. Don't attempt to eat only raw food for a period of time until you have cleansed the kidneys, liver, small intestines and colon. (See chapter 3 – Detoxification) Raw food and cooked food require different digestive enzymes, so they should not be mixed. Always eat the salad first as a starter, followed by the cooked food, rather than all mixed up together. This makes a difference in assimilation and helps increase the metabolism.

12. Women tend in general to have slower metabolisms than men. Around the menopausal years, the metabolism suddenly slows down even more, so more care is needed in the later years not to overeat and more attention needs to be paid to diet and lifestyle. At this time, it also becomes more difficult to lose weight but by following the dietary principles and exercising on a daily basis, we can increase detoxification and improve assimilation and metabolism. A sedentary lifestyle will slow down the metabolism and increase weight gain. If you eat too much and don't exercise enough, the food will be stored as fat.

13. Carbohydrates are energy foods, but we need to eat them in small quantities and eat the right kind of carbohydrates. Many people eat far too many carbohydrates. Fiber is necessary to keep the bowels working well but too much has a bloating and blocking effect and can cause constipation. Avoid refined carbohydrates such as white bread, white flour and cakes and biscuits, which create mucous and choose instead unrefined carbohydrates such as fruit, vegetables, wholegrain bread, basmati rice, lentils, chickpeas, oats, semolina, couscous, millet and barley. Eating too much bread or too many sandwiches can make you feel dull and lethargic. Bread is also known to be one of the highest allergens and is acidic. Both wheat and yeast are known to trigger allergic reactions. Most allergies are associated with too many toxins in the digestive tract. Toasted brown bread is more digestible. If you have difficulty digesting bread, substitute with rice crackers or rye crackers, which will also help reduce acidity.

Kitcheri is a highly nutritious Indian dish made with ghee and two parts rice and one part mung dhal, to which any of the following spices may be added, turmeric, cumin, fresh ginger, coriander, fennel and black pepper. Kitcheri is a complete protein and very balancing and good for the digestion. It is recommended to eat kitcheri twice a week or more.

14. Increase the amount of water rich foods that you eat and include regular helpings of fruit and vegetables, which provide fiber. Water rich foods contain a high content of chlorophyll, vitamins and minerals.

15. It is important to include the sweet taste in your diet, but sweets, pastries and biscuits, which contain white flour and white sugar, dull the mind and clog the body. Chocolate in particular is known to make the brain hazy and causes headaches when eaten in excess and it is addictive. Research has shown a connection between sugar and the degeneration of the cells and ageing. Too much sugar stresses the pancreas and lowers the immune system and cause

imbalances in the nervous system, which can lead to cravings and addictions.

Include soaked raisins, apricots, dates, figs and prunes regularly in your diet to satisfy the sweet taste, this will also prevent cravings for unhealthy sweets, chocolates and biscuits. Choose natural sweeteners such as honey, maple syrup, date syrup, molasses, carob syrup, rosewater, brown sugar and rock sugar. Don't use artificial sweeteners, most of them contain aspartame, which is damaging for the brain.

16. Select from a variety of foods, too much of any one food can have an adverse effect. Try to include all six tastes in your diet, sweet, sour, salty, bitter, astringent and pungent, this creates a balancing effect and helps prevent food cravings.

17. Give the body a rest once a week, choose one day a week to eat only fresh fruit or to drink fresh juices or to eat only soup.

18. Be aware when you eat, keep your attention on the food and chew your food properly, digestion begins in the mouth. If you talk, read or watch television whilst eating, your attention is not on the food and you will not chew properly and eat too fast or overeat. Don't eat when you are upset, this produces acidity, instead drink hot water with lemon and add honey when it has cooled down, this is soothing to the nervous system and then eat when you feel calmer.

19. Avid all frozen and tinned foods, they are old food, which contain no prana or life force energy. Always eat freshly prepared and freshly cooked foods; never eat leftovers, which are dead food and full of bacteria. Avoid any foods that contain chemicals, additives and colourings. Avoid using microwave ovens, which have been linked with cancer producing rays. Microwaves literally kill the food. Keep children away from microwave ovens, also pregnant women to protect the foetus.

20. Avid stimulants, which irritate the nervous system especially cigarettes, coffee, black tea and alcohol. Too much wine, coffee, black tea and fizzy drinks draw calcium from the bones and interfere with iron absorption. Coffee is very dehydrating and inhibits the absorption of vitamins and minerals and destroys vitamin B and C. Instead of coffee drink coffee substitutes such as Sonna, Bambu, Dandelion coffee or Raya's cup, an Ayurvedic coffee substitute. Instead of black tea, drink herbal teas or green tea.

21. Keep alcohol to a minimum. Alcohol is classed as a depressant and is known to kill brain cells. Yogis consider that alcohol lowers the vibrations of the subtle body and has a detrimental effect on the nervous system. Alcohol gives a high and low effect, first it stimulates the nervous system, then it depresses it, hence the foggy, heavy feeling the next morning after drinking alcohol. It induces low quality, drugged sleep and affects memory. Alcohol also causes cellular dehydration and is a trigger for many allergies and is known to weaken sperm and ovum.

22. Too much salt is one of the major causes of high blood pressure, it irritates the nervous system and deadens the taste buds and then you crave more salt. Use sea salt or herbal salts in moderation instead of regular salt. Add a little salt to cooking if you like but don't put extra salt on your food, it is easier to absorb when it is used in cooking. Use herbs and spices to flavour food instead.

23. Avoid cooking in aluminium pots, use stainless steel or earthenware instead. Aluminium from the pots can seep into the food and has a poisonous effect on the body.

24. Avoid genetically modified food and ask your local supermarket to label foods that have been genetically modified and to increase organic produce instead.

25. As much as possible avoid taking chemical antibiotics, which are known to depress the immune system and are often unnecessary but given routinely by many doctors. Use natural antibiotics such as

lapacho (pau d'arco) and take Ayurvedic, herbal or homeopathic remedies instead. If you do have to take antibiotics, do not take fruit juices, cola drinks or alcohol including wine whilst taking them, these can counteract the effect and be especially careful of any medicine that contains penicillin, which may cause an allergic reaction.

26. We need some fats in our diet, but we need to eat the right sort of fat. Cook with ghee and olive oil, which are the healthiest fats and the most nutritive substances for cooking. Try to take one or two teaspoons of ghee every day and at least one tablespoon of olive oil. Ghee and olive oil oleate the skin and digestive tract and prevent the bones from becoming brittle.

27. Avoid fermented and picked foods including vinegars and alcohol, which are considered tamasic and make the mind dull and are not good for the bones because of their high acidity levels. The exception to this is cider vinegar, which can be used instead.

28. Garlic, onions, eggplant, chillies, coffee, tea and alcohol are all considered rajasic because they have an agitating effect on the nervous system. Eggplant (aubergines) should never be given to children.

29. Before eating, verbally or silently give thanks for the food you are about to receive. Ask for the food to be blessed so that it may nourish your mind and body. Remember those that are less fortunate and do not have the luxury of eating good nutritious food every day.

Eating a Vegetarian Diet

There is enough scientific evidence available to verify that eating a nutritious, vegetarian diet is highly beneficial for your health. Animal products are high in saturated fats, which create high levels of cholesterol that can lead to heart disease. If you want to protect your heart, keep red meat to a minimum, or better still cut it out altogether. Nitrates, which are carcinogenic, are widely used in meat products. Meat also contains high levels of uric acid, which creates stones in the kidneys and bladder and is damaging for the bones and one of the causes of arthritis.

We do not need to eat meat for strength, the strongest animals are buffalo and elephants and they don't eat meat. Our teeth, jaws and digestive system are not designed to eat meat, which is the most difficult food for the body to digest and therefore results in fatigue, premature ageing and disease. Meat is filled with chemicals, hormones and preservatives and often contains parasites and worms, which can cause cancer and tumours and are not destroyed in cooking. Animals are regularly given large doses of penicillin and other drugs, which are harmful for humans.

Many gynaecologists now agree that the huge rise in hormone problems which so many women now face as well as infertility problems have a lot to do with the high level of hormones in meat and milk. Cows for instance are injected with bovine growth hormone so as to increase their milk production by 20%. This is thought to cause malignancy of the human breast. Many theories are currently being investigated into the connection between hormones in meat and milk and breast and uterine cancer.

If you eat fish or chicken, be choosy about the source. Shellfish especially are known to cause highly allergic reactions. Also be careful of where you buy your eggs and try to buy free-range eggs. The salmonella bacteria, which is found in eggs seems to be on the increase, it is very unpleasant and difficult to get rid of from the body.

Being vegetarian does not necessarily mean that a person is healthy, it is not enough just to cut out meat, you have to also adopt a healthy diet. For radiant health, you need to eat a wide variety of healthy foods including many of the superfoods and to incorporate the principles of balanced nutrition.

Kinesiology and Food

Kinesiology is a unique system of muscle testing which enables us to communicate with the intelligence of the body. Kinesiology can be used to test many different things but it is probably the most well known for testing for food intolerances and allergies. When the body is toxic or there are energy blockages, we may have allergic reactions to different substances. This often shows up on the skin through rashes, irritation, itching, blotches, swelling, excess heat, headaches, diarrhoea or nausea.

Kinesiology can identify many of these intolerances and allergens. Although a food may be generally good for you, you may at present have an imbalance or be toxic and so the body cannot tolerate a certain food at this time. Often this may be a food that you eat regularly and suddenly your body stats to react to it. We sometimes crave foods that the body cannot tolerate. This is seen in addictions. Intolerances are a reaction to something that the body cannot tolerate at this point in time. An allergic reaction is a much stronger reaction and could be harmful. Food sensitivity is a hidden factor behind many illnesses.

When I test people for food intolerance or allergens, I often find they are also very acidic or toxic and this is what lies behind the reaction. Detoxification is an important factor where there is food sensitivity or an allergic reaction. The most common food intolerances are caused by wheat, dairy products (lactose intolerance to milk or cheese) alcohol especially red wine, shell fish, chocolate, orange juice and strawberries.

Food intolerances may change or improve over a period of time or even from season to season and you may find that after changing your diet or after regular detoxification that you can then tolerate a substance that previously caused you a problem. It does not mean that because you are intolerant or allergic to a substance now that it will always be the case. For this reason, it is helpful to learn how to test yourself through Kinesiology. Through self-testing, you can find out, which foods, drinks, herbs, oils or supplements would be the best for you at any given time. Remember that you are a unique individual and that no two people respond in exactly the same way.

A recipe to make ghee

Ghee is simple to make. Buy two to three packets of unsalted butter. Cut the butter into cubes or slices and put it in a pan (preferably not aluminium), as soon as the butter starts to bubble, turn it down onto a very low heat. Simmer it for about fifteen minutes, but watch it to make sure it does not burn. Skim off the white froth, the milk solids, which come to the surface. Then take the ghee off the heat and allow it to cool, some white solids will also sink to the bottom of the pan. Before the ghee becomes cold and solidifies, sieve the ghee (the yellow liquid) through a muslin cloth and into a clean jar or container.

If you keep the ghee in the fridge, it becomes hard, if it is kept out of the fridge, it remains liquid. Take a tablespoon of ghee with your food every day, add it during or after cooking or spread it on toast.

3 - DETOXIFICATION

Detoxification is an essential part of any effective health regime, without it regeneration and rejuvenation cannot take place. The body needs regular detoxification in order to cleanse and increase the elimination of bacteria, toxins and wastes. This is well known in all systems of natural medicine and is recommended as a preventative measure for maintaining radiant health. In Ayurvedic clinics all over the world, people go for a special detoxification therapy called Pancha Karma. This includes daily oil massages, special herbal sweat boxes for detoxification, enemas, cleansing with ghee and oil, one day of fasting and a light, Ayurvedic diet. Many naturopathic clinics and spas offer similar therapies, some are more inclined towards beauty and relaxation, whereas others offer deeper cleansing and detoxification programmes. Unfortunately most of these treatments are very expensive and not within the budget of the average person, there is however a lot that you can do for yourself at home. The guidelines for different detoxification and cleansing programmes are given below.

The body cannot build new healthy cells and tissues or sufficiently absorb vital nutrients without first effectively detoxifying wastes. Cellular rejuvenation depends upon cellular detoxification and the body's ability to do the necessary repair work. The organs of elimination, the skin, lungs, liver, kidneys and colon need to be cleansed regularly in order to function effectively. Over the years, through incorrect diet, overeating, lack of exercise, slow metabolism or insufficient elimination, the body becomes clogged with a toxic layer; in Ayurveda this is called ama. Ama is a sticky waste that starts to build up in the digestive tract, in the colon and intestines, it then moves upwards and circulates throughout the body. Ama can be found in any part of the body, even in the brain, it clogs the channels of circulation, thickens the blood and restricts the flow of nutrients to the cells and organs.

If you have eaten a lot of processed foods, meat and dairy most likely you will have a lot of ama. By changing one's diet and eating more cleansing foods like fresh fruit, salads and vegetables and regularly fasting for one day a week, then gradually the body can be cleansed and the ama can be removed.

Symptoms of a build up of ama include a coated tongue in the mornings, stiff joints, backache, dullness, foggy mind, low energy, low immunity, body odour, skin problems and allergies. If toxins are not sufficiently eliminated, this can result in an overload and eventually create a crisis. Toxicity causes a lack of vitality, extreme fatigue, stagnation, weakening of the immune system, premature ageing and disease. When there is a lot of ama in the body and the immune system becomes depleted, it is easy for infections and viruses to take hold. Detoxification helps improve immunity.

Excess waste and toxic matter cause a strain on the liver and kidneys and block the intestines and arteries and increase weight gain, which can put pressure on the heart. Many people overeat which blocks the digestive and eliminative systems. Everyone can benefit from giving the digestive system a rest once a week and by cutting out foods, which are hard to digest such as meat, hard cheeses, junk food, processed foods and left over foods, which are dead food.

Agni, the digestive power and fire element in the body plays an important part in detoxification and needs to be well balanced. If agni is too weak, then there will not be enough fire to digest the food properly and this causes congestion and a build up of ama and weight gain. If agni is too strong, it will create too much heat and this can cause ulcers, sores and inflammation. Spices can increase the fire element and digestive power in the body. You can improve a sluggish digestive system by adding spices to your food, choose from fresh ginger, black pepper, cumin, coriander and turmeric.

The process of aging is seen in some traditions as unnatural and in countries like India and Tibet, there are masters over a hundred years old and in very good health. Ageing occurs when the body is unable to regenerate and repair to the degree that is needed because deterioration is happening at a faster rate than the body can cope with. Certainly with the right attention and care and including regular detoxification, we can prevent premature ageing by paying attention to our habits and lifestyle. Everything we do affects our health and well-being and therefore has its consequences. We need to change unhealthy and destructive habits, which cause degeneration and take more care of ourselves so that regeneration can occur. Your thoughts on this will also affect the outcome, if you expect to age fast you will, if you expect to regenerate you will. This doesn't mean that at seventy, you will look twenty, it means that at any age, you can sustain a high level of energy, maintain your strength and flexibility and have a clear and creative mind, which enables you to do the things you want to do and to continue to enjoy life to the full.

One of the major factors in all degenerative diseases is the accumulation of toxic matter in the organs, tissues and cells. Circulation then becomes impaired and congestion and stagnation occur. Toxic accumulation creates digestive problems, including bloating, bad breath, constipation, frequent diarrhoea, skin problems, allergies, smelly stools, yeast infections, frequent colds and an overproduction of urine or sweat as the body tries to eliminate. Then problems may develop in the muscles, the bones, the reproductive system and the immune system.

According to Ayurveda, one of the root causes of many diseases starts with toxicity in the digestive tract from undigested food and other substances that leave residues in the body including harmful chemicals, medicines, mercury from fillings, dyes and colourings, additives, hormones, pesticides, fungus, air pollutants, allergens and water pollution. Mercury, which is a component in amalgam fillings, is one of the most toxic metals and has been banned in Sweden, Finland, Germany and Canada. Mercury can leak into the body and cause poisoning and has been linked to chronic fatigue, MS and Alzheimer's. It is recommended to remove all amalgam fillings.

Ama, undigested food and toxic substances create putrefaction in the body and often cannot be eliminated due to over congestion. A polluted intestinal track creates unclean, toxic blood that impairs the proper functioning of the liver and the kidneys and affects metabolism and can create a chemical imbalance, which affects the cellular level. This results in poor digestion, sluggishness, low energy, fatigue and weight gain. Too much toxic waste matter in the intestines is a breeding ground for parasites, fungus, bacteria and worms. High toxicity levels and the accumulation of toxic wastes combined with the body's inability to detoxify sufficiently can result in cysts and tumours and are a major contributing factor in cancerous growths and cellular deformation. Everyone needs to promote better functioning of the organs and to improve digestion, assimilation and elimination.

The gastrointestinal tract is the food channel; it is one very long tube. It starts in the mouth, goes down to the stomach, to the small intestines, colon and anus. This channel needs to be kept clean and regularly detoxified so that ama in this region can be removed. The tongue gives a good indication as to the internal state of the body specifically the digestive system. Any discolouration of the tongue or coating on the tongue or ulcers, sore gums, tooth decay or bad breath indicate problems in this area. Everything that is taken into the body has to go through the process of digestion, assimilation and elimination. Through assimilation the cells are nourished and whatever is not useful is then eliminated. Nutrients are absorbed through the intestinal walls into the bloodstream.

The main organs of elimination are the skin, the lungs, the liver, the kidneys and the colon. These organs must be kept in the best working order for them to do their work properly. Sluggish organs will not be able to eliminate sufficiently and then a toxic build up can occur, hence the need for regular detoxification. How efficiently the body is able to eliminate wastes is one of the main keys to good health. This is more difficult if you are overweight because the body has more to cope with. When you are stressed or overtired, the body has to use extra energy to support the nervous system and cannot detoxify properly.

The skin is the largest organ of detoxification. Where there is an excess of toxins, the body will try to expel them through the skin. The condition of your skin is a reflection of what is happening inside the body. Skin problems are related to incorrect diet, stress, bowel problems, sluggish or toxic liver or the body's inability to detoxify sufficiently. Debris and toxins are constantly released through the skin; therefore it is essential to keep the skin as clean as possible. The same attention you pay to your face, you should pay to your whole body including your feet. If you try going for a few days without using a deodorant and there is a strong body odour, this will tell you that you need to detoxify.

Make sure to have a shower or bath every morning to rinse off the toxins and debris that have been eliminated during the night, this is basic hygiene; otherwise they will be reabsorbed back into the skin again. One third of all wastes are eliminated through the skin. The main detoxification takes place between 10pm and 2am, so if you have a lot of late nights, you miss the opportunity for maximum detoxification to take place. Before showering take a few minutes to exfoliate the skin with a soft, natural brush or loofah to slough off dead cells, increase circulation and to keep the uppermost layer of the skin free from debris. This removes dead cells and wastes that might clog the pores and helps eliminate cellulite, which is a build up of toxic substances due to insufficient lymph drainage. The skin of your face also needs daily exfoliation with a very soft brush or natural exfoliant. As you get older, metabolic changes slow down the release of dead cells and we need more exfoliation. It is also recommended to lightly oil the body before showering with sesame oil. It only takes about five minutes to do both, but if you don't have enough time, then alternate with exfoliating one day and massaging the next.

Detoxifying the skin through the therapeutic use of water and healing baths can be traced back as far as the Essene teachings and ancient Greece. The term spa evolved from these ancient practices and originally meant a place where the water had special healing properties because of a high mineral content, which could both detoxify and heal the body from certain ailments. There are some special places where there are hot or cold water springs where the water is said to be very healing. The modern day spas are based upon the same premise and use hydrotherapy and thalassatherapy and often include seaweed treatments or mud therapies, which were known to many indigenous tribes such as the native American Indians and the Aborigines who used the earth for detoxification and healing.

The Dead Sea is well known for having the highest concentration of minerals in the world and thousands of people go to spas in the area to heal skin problems. Dead Sea salts and Dead Sea black mud are very therapeutic both for drawing out toxins and for relieving muscular pain and stress. Steam baths or Turkish baths are wonderful for deep cleansing and are considered preferable to saunas because of the effect of the steam on the pores. To improve the condition of your skin and to detoxify the skin, either have a weekly Turkish bath or sauna or therapeutic baths at home. If you have high blood pressure, heart problems, hot flushes or a lot of heat in your body, do not have heat treatments or hot baths.

The most powerful of all baths as a general detoxifier is a bath with Chaparrel, which is one of the favourite herbs of the American Indians. It detoxifies the blood, kidneys, liver and lymph and stimulates the thymus. It is an antioxidant and antiviral and is recommended in the treatment of viruses, flu, herpes, rheumatism, arthritis and cancer. The way to prepare a Chaparrel bath is to make a tea by boiling 2-3 tablespoons of the herb in approximately a litre of water, bring to the boil and then simmer for five minutes. Then strain the concoction and add it to the bath water. Stay in the bath for 20-30 minutes and after the bath, lie down and relax for a while, this is a very powerful treatment. Weekly Chaparrel baths should be taken as part of a detoxifying treatment for a period of four to six weeks and then repeated again after three months.

You can then continue having weekly Dead Sea salt baths to which you can add one drop of juniper oil, which has been dissolved in a little sesame or olive oil. Epsom salts and magnesium salts in the bath also help eliminate toxins. Warm water is very relaxing and helps release tension from the body as well as helping the minerals from the salts to be absorbed into the body. You can add a little oil to the bath, preferably sesame, olive or almond oil to prevent dryness. When it is cold or you feel chilled, you can add three drops of ginger oil diluted in carrier oil to the water. Footbaths are also very beneficial especially after a tiring day; add one tablespoon of Dead Sea salts to the water and the minerals will be absorbed through the feet. Putting the feet in a mud bath also helps draw out the toxins. Baths are more beneficial and relaxing for the whole body and especially the nervous system. You can also add different essential oils to the bath but remember to always dilute them in a carrier oil otherwise they may burn the skin.

Many nature cures are based on water cures. Drinking lots of water can eliminate many illnesses and diseases. Most people are dehydrated because of not drinking enough water or not eating enough water rich foods like fruit and vegetables and because of drinking too much coffee and tea, which dehydrates the body and makes them acidic. Lack of sufficient water intake can cause premature ageing, wrinkles, dry skin, constipation, headaches, arthritis, kidney stones, lymph, urinary, kidney and bladder problems. Water deficiency can also cause congestion, constipation and depression. It is essential to drink enough water, at least six glasses a day. Do not drink ice-cold water or add ice to your drinks because it puts out the digestive fire.

The body needs enough water to keep the blood clean and pure and to flush toxins and accumulated wastes from the cells and tissues through the bloodstream to the kidneys. The accumulation of toxic wastes and excess acidity cause the thickening of the blood. Acidic foods include coffee, tea, alcohol, meat, cheese and pickled and fermented foods. Drinking enough water and detoxifying the kidneys helps improve the quality of the blood. The kidneys are the master filters of the body and these filters need to be kept clean. The kidneys control water metabolism including the absorption of water and break down urea, uric acid, hormones, vitamins and salts and flush out toxins and chemicals through the urine. The kidneys also maintain the correct PH balance. High levels of acidity cause an imbalance in the urinary system and result in cystitis, cellulite, premature aging and degenerative diseases such as arthritis, rheumatism and osteoporosis. It is recommended to do kidney cleansing at least twice a year.

The colon, (the large intestine) excretes wastes that cannot be used by the body, it also absorbs water. Where there is a lack of water in the body, this can produce dryness in the colon resulting in constipation, dry skin, allergies and many other symptoms. To maintain good health, it is necessary to keep the colon clean. Over the years, the colon becomes clogged through an accumulation of toxic matter and undigested food, which can form a hard crust on the lining of the colon. This narrows the colon and makes elimination more difficult and impairs the proper absorption of nutrients. There is also an important connection between the colon and the bones, if the colon is blocked, the absorption of calcium is prevented and this will affect the bones. Stagnated faeces in the colon leads to a build up of wastes (ama) in the rest of the body.

Colonic irrigation (also known as colon hydrotherapy) is an effective way of removing wastes from the colon. Filtered, warm water is pumped into the colon several times, and at first the inner part of the colon is cleaned and then the water peels off the layers of toxic, crusted matter from the walls of the colon and releases it. One of the reasons that people cannot lose weight is because the waste removal systems of the body are not working efficiently enough. Unless the colon is clean and wastes can pass through the colon unimpeded, any other methods of cleansing such as juicing, fasting, or herbal formulas cannot be truly effective. It is advisable to clean the colon and kidneys first before attempting any other cleansing programmes. Don't think of doing liver or intestinal cleansing until this has been done, otherwise you will be loading the system with more toxic stuff, which it cannot get rid of. Colonic irrigation will help rectify problems of constipation, diarrhoea, headaches, skin problems, allergies, parasites and help with weight problems. It can also help relieve spasms of the bowel and lower back pain. After the colon has been cleansed, the therapist may recommend reflorastation, a simple implant of healthy bacteria to bring the body back to balance if the natural bacterial flora has been disturbed or is not sufficient.

After the colon has been cleansed, you can then take regular weekly enemas. Enemas are considered to have tremendous therapeutic value in Ayurveda. Although the enema is inserted into the anus, it is said to be able to draw impurities from all parts of the body including the feet and head. This is very evident in people who suffer headaches and after taking an enema their headache disappears. Enemas are also very settling for the nervous system especially unctuous (oil) enemas. There are different kinds of enemas, water, herbal, coffee and unctuous. Many people balk at the idea of taking an enema, this is only because it is something unknown to them. I discovered an old herbal remedies book, which was written in 1903 and was surprised to find that the author recommended regular enemas for the relief of pain and congestion, even back then, the value of enemas was known. Once you come to realize the benefits of regular enemas, you will want to include them as a part of your detoxification routine.

Always use a clean empty enema bag, which has nothing in it, don't use chemical or prepared enema solutions. It is best to use room temperature water for the enema, which has been boiled and allowed to cool. When you insert the nozzle of the enema use a little natural cream or vasoline so as to feel more comfortable and lie on your right side so the water can travel up the descending part of the colon and across the transverse colon. You may need to evacuate soon after introducing the water in which case do the enema again, you want to try to hold the water in the body for 10 to 15 minutes. Different herbs such as Neem (an Indian herb) for blood purification or Dandelion for cleansing or Camomile for soothing can be added. Add about one teaspoon of herbs to the boiled water, boil for about five minutes and then strain before putting in the enema bag. If there is too much heat in the body, take cool (not cold) enemas.

It is good to alternate between water and unctuous enemas. An oil enema can be made by mixing equal amounts of ghee, sesame oil and honey, half a cup is enough. More oil can be used for chronic constipation but colonics would be recommended first. Unctuous enemas oil the body from inside and are very good for dry skin. In hot weather, take unctuous enemas in the evening.

Coffee enemas need a special mention. People are often astounded when I tell them to do a coffee enema, but they have remarkable effects. Drinking coffee irritates the nervous system and membranes and causes acidity but coffee enemas have a totally different effect because the coffee does not pass through the digestive system. The caffeine causes dilation of the bile ducts, which facilitates the excretion of toxic matter, promotes bile flow, stimulates the liver, releases toxic residues, counteracts inflammation and relieves pain. Coffee enemas are helpful in all degenerative diseases including cancer. Coffee enemas also help with allergies, depression, restlessness and sleeplessness, for these symptoms it is best to do a coffee enema in the evening. Clinical practice in various clinics and centres has shown that a coffee enema is effective even with severe pain and is well tolerated by most patients.

To make a coffee enema, add 3 tablespoons of ground, coffee (Greek coffee is best) to 16 ounces of water, (about two large mugs) bring to the boil and then simmer for 10 minutes, allow to cool and then filter twice through a fine strainer. It is advisable to do a water enema first as you may need to evacuate quickly and lose the effects of the coffee enema. Then do the coffee enema and try to keep it in the body for 10-15 minutes. It is recommended to do coffee enemas once or twice a month or more often if needed.

The liver is a very large organ, which has many functions. The liver aids digestion, circulation and metabolism, blood formation and coagulation, it detoxifies, cleans the blood, destroys old blood cells and removes poisonous substances, it forms bile and stores vital nutrients including proteins and glycogen. The liver is one of the few organs, which has the ability to regenerate itself but when the liver fails, the body dies. Allergic reactions are linked to toxicity of the liver. There is also a connection between toxicity of the liver and addictions to food, drugs and alcohol. Excessive alcohol weakens the liver and impedes its function.

Regular liver detoxification is vital to maintain and support maximum liver function and is recommended as a part of any natural health programme. Detoxification of the liver is a two-step process, first the toxins are made water-soluble and then they are eliminated. It is not recommended to do liver cleansing when the weather is very hot. Before doing a liver cleanse, first cleanse the kidneys and the colon. There are different ways to do a liver cleanse, there are various herbal formulas that can be taken or stronger purges, which release liver and gall bladder stones.

The quality of the blood affects the health of your body, it is important to have clean, thin blood. Kidney, liver and colon cleanses help purify the blood. Thick or acidic blood affects the arteries and causes degenerative diseases. The quality of the blood is affected by the amount of water you drink, lack of water creates dehydration and thick blood.

Massage and reflexology are valuable treatments, which aid detoxification. Almost every woman enjoys the benefits of a massage. There are many different types of massage; all massage is helpful in stimulating the circulation. Deep therapeutic massage removes tension from the muscles, whereas aromatherapy massage with the use of essential oils is more relaxing and balancing.

Ayurveda recommends the benefits of giving yourself a daily massage. This only takes a couple of minutes. Cold pressed sesame oil is the best oil for detoxification. Sesame oil contains the largest amount of linoleic acid, which is antibiotic, antifungal, antiflammatory and antioxidant and can halt the growth of cancer cells. Current research is being done on the use of sesame oil on skin cancer and other forms of cancer. Make sure to use cold pressed sesame oil, not the sesame oil, which is used for cooking. Before use, the sesame oil needs to be cured. Warm the oil on a low heat, add a couple of drops of water and when it starts to crackle, it is ready, do not allow it to boil. Whilst doing your daily massage, remember to give special attention to the abdominal area, this will help release gas and bloatedness and improve intestinal function. It can also release deep stress, which is held in the abdominal area. Work clockwise, around the navel, make several circles starting with small ones and then larger ones. This can also be done lying down as a way to release tension whilst breathing deeply.

Massage with sesame oil all over the body for a couple of minutes and then shower, don't use soap except on your private parts and then pat your body try, this leaves a very thin film of sesame oil on the body which will be absorbed through the pores during the day. Whenever you have more time, such as weekends, leave the oil on for ten to thirty minutes as a deeper treatment and then follow it by a warm bath, which will help the pores open and absorb the oil. Over a period of time, you will see a big difference in your skin; it will be soft and silky. Also do a head massage with sesame oil every week before washing your hair and leave the oil on for 30 minutes. Sesame oil can also be used in the mouth to prevent mouth and gum problems. Swirl around one teaspoon of oil in the mouth and then spit it out and repeat again. Also rub a little sesame oil or ghee in each nostril and inhale, this lubricates the nose and the sinuses and helps clear mucus. The nose is the doorway to the brain and by sniffing sesame oil or ghee up the nose it can also help clear mental stress. Maintenance of the nostrils is considered to be an essential yogic practice as the nostrils are the outlets of two major nadis, (energy channels) which nourish the brain.

Castor oil has become famous through the work of Edgar Cayce; he called castor oil the miracle curer and recommended castor oil packs for cysts, tumours, breast lumps, bowel diseases and almost anything. Layers of cloth soaked in castor oil are placed on the part of the body where there is a problem with a warming pad on top for about half an hour to one hour every day for as long as necessary.

Manual Lymphatic Drainage is a very gentle massage with specific semi-circular movements, which stretch the skin and open the lymphatic vessels under the skin. This allows greater amounts of metabolic waste products and excess water to be removed from the tissues. MLD reduces lymphatic congestion, fluid retention and cellulite and is especially recommended for lymphoedema and obesity.

Reflexology is one of the most popular alternative therapies today. It can be seen as a general maintenance programme for both the mind and body and is a very valuable therapy on its own or in assisting any detoxification programme. Through stimulating the nerve endings and the reflex points of the feet, the whole body is stimulated. Reflexology increases the circulation of the blood and lymph and helps release toxins and wastes from the liver, kidneys and intestines. It strengthens all the body systems and improves digestion, elimination and metabolism. It also balances the hormones, boosts the immune system and creates a state of homeostasis.

Ear coning is an ancient process that was used in India, China, Tibet, Egypt and American Indian cultures to cleanse the upper lymphatic system including the ears, the sinuses and eustachian tubes. Many doctors in America have switched from irrigation techniques to ear coning. In Germany doctors are taught ear coning as a part of their training. Ear coning removes wax, fungus and candida from the upper tract. It clears the eustachian tubes and sinuses, helps with earaches, headaches, sore throats, lung congestion and clears the mind. It is useful for smokers who are trying to give up smoking or for people who have been heavy smokers.

Many natural therapists now practise ear coning and use traditional cones made by Hopi Indians. These are very long and made from pure cotton, dipped in beeswax and different combinations of herbs; they are made according to the lunar cycle. There are ear cones in the market that are not made in the traditional way, which are not so good as they do not contain herbs. It is recommended to do at least one or two ear coning sessions a year, more if necessary, to keep the nasal, sinuses and upper lymphatic tract clear. Although the ear cones are used nowadays mainly for physical detoxification, they have other benefits too. The ancient Egyptians used them to improve brain function and to aid concentration, improve memory and increase the activity of the pineal and pituitary glands. The process is painless and relaxing and children can benefit too. Many people who have had constant earache or sinus problems find they get instant relief.

Guidelines for Detoxification Programmes

After reading the previous section, you will have understood how important detoxification is both for the maintenance of radiant health and also as a prevention of imbalances and illness. Prevention is always better than cure. When we regularly detoxify the body, we give the organs the opportunity to improve their function and strengthen the immune system. Detoxification is an on-going process, not something you do once or twice and then forget about. There needs to be regular, thorough and efficient elimination of wastes and toxins from the cells, tissues and the blood.

When doing any detoxification programme, always listen to your intuition and to your body as to what is right for you, if in doubt consult with an Ayurvedic practitioner or a naturopath who can give you more individual attention. The most important thing to remember is to go slowly and not to try to make too many changes at once. When you do any sort of cleansing, there may be a healing reaction as the body starts to throw out toxic stuff. You might experience headaches, bad breathe, heavily coated tongue, intestinal discomfort, diarrhoea, pain, skin rashes or spots, itching, tiredness and strong smelling urine or perspiration as poisons and pollutants are released from the tissues and organs. These symptoms usually clear up within a few days, you don't want to stop the healing reaction, you want the toxins to clear out of your body, but if the symptoms are too strong slow down your detoxification programme or get advice from a natural health practitioner. If there is pain anywhere in the body, the fastest relief can usually be attained through taking a coffee enema.

You may not have any of these symptoms; it is just good to know about them, should they occur.

The following are general guidelines for detoxification programmes:

Upon rising, before cleaning your teeth always clean your tongue with a stainless steel tongue scraper; this will give an indication of the toxicity level. Make this a daily habit, if you don't clean your tongue, the toxins go back down your throat. After cleaning your teeth, floss your teeth and use a natural mouthwash. To make your own natural mouth wash, add 2 drops tea tree oil, 1 drop myrrh oil and 1 drop of lavender oil to warm water and rinse, this prevents infections of the mouth and gums. Sniff a little ghee or sesame oil up each nostril. Take a few minutes to exfoliate and oil your body as indicated previously.

Start the day by drinking a cup of warm water, with one teaspoon of lemon and one teaspoon of honey or one of cider vinegar and one of honey. Lemon has a cooling effect on the body and cider vinegar a heating effect, both are cleansing. Throughout the day, drink lots of hot water with a few slices of fresh ginger, hot water has a cleansing effect and ginger stimulates the digestion fire.

Follow the water with 1-2 tablespoons of aloe vera juice. Aloe vera can be taken up to two to three times a day, before food. It has countless benefits. It is antiviral, antifungal, antibacterial and antioxidant. It helps with assimilation and metabolism. First it flushes out the toxins, helps clean the digestive tract and heals disorders of the bowel including inflamed bowel, colitis, diverculosis, irritable bowel, constipation and diarrhoea. It cleans the colon, detoxifies the blood and lymphatic system. After cleansing, it heals the epithelial tissue including damaged skin in the lining of the gut, bronchial tubes, genital tract, bladder, arteries and capillaries. It is also said to be helpful in arthritis, asthma, ME, lupus and immune system diseases, chronic back pain, rheumatoid and osteoarthritis.

Aloe vera can also be used directly on the skin in the form of a gel to help acne, eczema, psoriasis, ulcers, burns, skin problems, stings and bites. Aloe vera is renowned for its power to soothe and heal. It can be taken separately or if you don't like the taste, it can be added to juice. Most aloe vera juices contain plant-based stabilizers and natural preservatives. If aloe vera makes your stools too loose, then take less. There are many different aloe vera juices on the market, try to find one that is not watery and contains a lot of sap.

Throughout the day, drink as much water as possible. Hot water is very cleansing, keep it in a thermos flask and sip it continuously throughout the day, this will help release ama. Drink bottled spring water unless you are lucky enough to live in an area where the water is pure. Tap water usually contains too much fluoride and lots of chemicals. Use water filters to wash your vegetables and for cooking.

There are several herbal teas that you can drink to support the eliminative process. Lapacho, also known as pao d'arco is a natural antibiotic and a powerful immune stimulant, it helps fight fungus, parasites, infections and candida and is a tonic for the liver in the elimination of wastes. Lapacho can be drunk on going and is good to take during the winter months for the prevention of colds and flu.

Dandelion is one of the most detoxifying and cleansing herbs in the plant kingdom; it can be drunk as a tea or added to salads. It assists the lymphatic system by increasing circulation and is a tonic for the liver and cleans the blood. There are also specific herbs and spices, which help purify the blood. The number one herb of the American Indians is Chaparrel, but it needs to be taken in very small amounts otherwise it can be toxic. Bitter greens and herbs are good including coriander, dill, basil and neem. Turmeric is an excellent blood cleanser and so is beetroot. Burdock assists the liver and helps kidney function, it is also good for dry, scaly skin and it helps dissolve lymphatic congestion and removes dead cells. Nettles and green juices are high in chlorophyll and promote blood cleansing. Liquorice, Indian sarsaparilla and Plantain are also blood cleansers. Fenugreek, celery and cabbage juice detoxify the lymph system.

71

Apples are powerful detoxifiers; they contain a high content of pectin, which is cleansing for the digestive system and the gall bladder. Try to eat an apple every day or to drink fresh apple juice. Stewed apples with soaked raisins, dried figs and prunes are good for breakfast, promote internal cleansing and give you lots of energy. Grapes are known for their special cleansing effects. Beetroot, celery, asparagus and kelp are cleansing for the bladder and the kidneys and stimulate urine flow.

Kelp, artichokes and green vegetables especially spinach help detoxify the liver. Chlorella is a green algae, which has amazing medicinal properties. It helps cleanse heavy metals and synthetics from the blood and the organs and cleanses the bowel, kidneys and liver. Chlorella causes the beneficial bacteria of the stomach (Lactobacillus) to multiply so as to protect against fungus and other bacteria.

It is good to do a PH test every couple of months to see if there is an excess of acidity. You can do this at home by buying litmus paper and urinating on it. The normal count is 7.2, lower shows acidity, if it is a lot lower than you must take some measures to counteract it. High acidity thickens the blood and affects the bones and causes arthritis and is a major factor in osteoporosis. Bacteria thrive in an acidic environment. Try to have a more alkaline diet and to avoid foods, which are highly acidic, these include cigarettes, tea, coffee and alcohol. Wheat and rye are also acidic; choose rice, barley and millet instead. The most alkaline fruits are apples, melons and grapes. Besides changing to a more alkaline diet, it is also advisable to do a kidney cleanse and drink noni juice, which helps balance the PH level and neutralizes and removes acids from the body.

Yeast, moulds and fungi along with toxins increase acidity and make the cells sick. High acidity causes pain and stiffness. Removing acids from the body increases the body's ability to absorb vitamins, minerals and protein.

Ghee is a very important substance in Ayurveda; it is both cleansing and nourishing. It oils the body from inside and prevents dryness and is very helpful for the digestive system. It is used in Ayurvedic clinics as part of a cleansing programme to release toxins from the digestive tract. (See the recipe on how to make ghee in Chapter 2 – Conscious Eating.)

An important part of detoxification is to regularly clean the organs. It is good to clean the kidneys first, the kidneys are the drains of the body and if the drains are blocked, then everything else blocks up too. It is recommended to cleanse the kidneys at least twice a year or more if necessary. There are many different combinations of kidney herbs that can be used, but the most effective that I have come across is one specific herb from the Amazon called quebra pedra. This herb is well known in Brazil, Peru, India and the Bahamas where it is known as the stonebreaker.

Thousands of tiny stones accumulate in the kidneys and gall bladder especially if you have been a tea or coffee drinker. Quebra pedra gradually breaks down all calcified deposits and stones and removes them. It is helpful for all kidney and urinary infections including cystitis and thrush and strengthens and fortifies the liver and gall bladder by stimulating bile production as well as improving lymphatic function. It acts as a diuretic, stimulating the elimination of uric acid. Quebra pedra should be drunk on-going for four to six weeks and then drunk a couple of times a week to maintain kidney and liver support and to keep the ureters clean. Drink plenty of water as well whilst doing a kidney cleanse to help flush out the toxins. Avoid drinking black tea or coffee whilst doing a kidney cleanse otherwise you are defeating the purpose; both black tea and coffee create stones in the kidneys.

You can do a colon cleanse at the same time as doing a kidney cleanse. It is recommended to have a colonics once or twice a year especially if you have a history of constipation or bowel problems.

After a kidney cleanse and colon cleanse, you can do a liver cleanse and cleanse the small intestines. Detoxifying and regenerating the liver is very important. Rio Super Detox is a combination of herbs specially prepared to detoxify the liver. It comes in the form of a tincture, which is taken for 20 days and can be repeated as often as needed or taken every three months to maintain and support regular liver function. It releases toxins, including metabolic wastes, bacteria, viruses, residues of pharmaceutical drugs, alcohol, food additives and other chemical pollutants. Rio Super Detox also contains milk thistle, which is known to be the best herb for regenerating the liver.

A build up of toxins and debris in the small intestines affects the proper absorption of food and this can result in malnutrition, skin problems, rashes and allergies. Taking a natural hypoallergenic fibre such as Rio Super Cleanse, which contains psyllium husks, herbs and lactobacillus cleanses the small intestines and colon by loosening old fecal matter and promoting healthy bowel function.

Triphala is an Ayurvedic formula, which is a synergy of Indian herbs. It is a mild laxative, which makes it a very good bowel cleanser as it detoxifies the body slowly. It clears ama and toxins from the digestive tract, the blood, muscle, fat tissues and other channels of the body. Triphala can be taken for 3-6 months at a time to remove ama from the digestive tract and other areas of the body.

Occasionally it is good to do a parasite cleanse, parasites can be at the root of many problems. Many people have problems in the intestinal tract, which they are unaware of including fungus, worms, and parasites, these can lead to chronic and degenerative diseases. Black walnut tincture is the best herb for parasite cleansing, this can be taken as a tincture for a month and can be taken in conjunction with any of the other cleanses.

Cleansing of the organs is recommended before attempting other detoxification processes or fasting, otherwise toxins will just circulate in the body and more waste will be dumped into an already polluted system and this will create more work for the liver and the kidneys.

After doing, kidney, colon, liver and small intestinal cleansing, you may wish to do deeper cleansing of the tissues, which is necessary for regeneration. The best way to start doing this is by giving your body a rest once a week. People who have not done any cleanses tend to be very toxic and if they try to fast even for a day they may get strong headaches, pain, skin eruptions, sleepiness, nervousness or other symptoms. It is important not to detoxify too fast, it is better to follow a gradual purification and cleansing programme, which everyone can benefit from. Never do any sort of fasting if you feel stressed, emotionally low or have a heavy workload.

Most people eat far too much food and this makes the body sluggish. An essential rule in conscious eating is not to ever overeat. Always leave the table feeling you could have eaten just a little more. We should only fill the stomach to two thirds of its capacity, leaving one third empty for proper assimilation to take place. Fasting one day a week is very beneficial for the body (after cleansing the organs), it gives the digestive system a rest and allows the body time to process and assimilate.

Fasting is recommended in many traditions as part of a spiritual discipline. (Don't do fasting if you are on medication or seriously ill unless recommended by a doctor or naturopath.) Juice fasting once a week, gives the body a rest and cleanses the blood. Apples are very cleansing for the digestive system. You can alternate with apple, carrot and green juices. Remember not to mix fruit with vegetables juices; the exception to this is apples. (See Conscious Eating for more information on juices.) If you do a juice fast, you must take a water enema in the evening, otherwise the toxins will continue to circulate in the body and be drawn back into the tissues. Enemas are essential in any fasting routine, whether you are doing a one day or three day fast or longer. You can drink hot water with a few slices of fresh ginger to which you can add 2 basil leaves, 2 mint leaves and 2 cloves to drink during the day. You can also drink dandelion tea and add a tablespoon of dandelion tea to the evening enema. When you are fasting, you need to take extra rest, make sure to be in bed by 10pm the latest. After fasting the taste buds become more refined so food tastes better. Fasting helps reduce cravings.

In cold climates or during winter you need more warming, nourishing foods. During cold periods if you find it difficult to drink only juices one day a week because of feeling cold or weak, instead you can eat homemade soup made from fresh vegetables. This is also suitable for people who have not previously done any detoxification programme. Soup is light on the stomach but does not have the cleansing effect of juices.

After you have done weekly juice fasts for a period of time and you feel comfortable and are not having any toxic reactions, then once a month, preferably around the period of full moon, you can do a three day juice fast. The energies are stronger at this time and this promotes deeper cleansing. Or you can try one day on juice and two days on vegetable soup. (Take enemas every evening.) Fasting is a powerful way to detoxify the tissues; it slows down the aging process and extends life. Fasting also has a profound effect on the mind, it becomes much clearer as debris is released from the brain and it can open you to spiritual experiences.

Green juices are very cleansing and nourishing, all bitter greens are cleansing. Longer fasts especially water fasts should only be done after you have done lots of cleanses and you definitely should not work if you are doing a longer fast as the body needs lots of rest when deep cleansing is going on and there may be healing reactions, so go slow. Always reintroduce heavier foods gradually.

Drinking fresh fruit juices and eating only fruit until lunchtime is a good practise especially during the summer months. Fruit gives natural energy. If your digestive fire is strong and you do not have any bowel problems, you might like to try a raw food diet for a few weeks during summer.

The healing power of grapes is known and recommended for many illnesses by naturopaths and in natural healing clinics all over the world. Many cancers including leukaemia have been treated with the grape cure. There is a simple grape fast that can be done at home for a month, which is very effective and easy to do. If you have cancer or any other serious degenerative disease, you should not attempt the grape fast alone but in a centre or clinic that specializes in such practises and under the guidance of a doctor.

Drink 24 ounces of freshly pressed dark grape juice throughout the morning, do not take anything else except water until lunchtime. Then eat a normal lunch and an early light dinner. Make sure not to overeat during this time and not to eat anything else after 8pm in the evening. This means that nothing is taken into the body for 16 hours, from 8pm until 12am the next day except grape juice. You can do this from two to four weeks once a year and it has a very healing effect.

Although this chapter has been addressing the physical level, we must remember that we also need to do mental and emotional detoxification, releasing negative thoughts and patterns and the suppression and holding of emotions. Everything is interlinked. Stress can affect any part of the body, the heart, digestion, metabolism, reproduction and the hormones. Distress on any level is registered in the body. Anger creates acids in the body and fear creates blockages and stagnation. If there is something that we cannot digest emotionally, it will interfere with our physical digestion. If there is something we cannot let go of or cannot release from the past, there may be difficulty with elimination or colon function. More information on the connection between the effects of the emotions on the physical body will be addressed in the chapters on healing.

Losing Weight

Overweight is a major concern of many women, especially as they get older. Conscious eating is very important and so are the dietary principles of balanced nutrition. It is not just what you eat but also how well you digest, assimilate and eliminate your food and how efficiently your metabolism functions. To lose weight you have to do it gradually without stress or discomfort. We put on weight gradually over the years; in the same way we can comfortably lose it by following all the advice given in conscious eating as well as regular detoxification.

Your body type also has an influence on whether you find it easy or not to lose weight. If you have a strong, well-built or muscular body you are never going to be thin so don't become obsessed about it. The aim is to reduce excess weight gradually, to feel good and remain healthy without getting stressed. Avoid going on crash diets, which don't work in the long run and make cravings worse.

To lose weight easily, cut out all sugar including alcohol and keep starchy foods to a minimum. Avoid overeating, emotional eating, eating in between meals and eating heavy meals late at night. Remember you also need to move your energy in order to increase your metabolism by exercising every day, walk daily for a minimum of thirty minutes and do some Yoga stretches daily. A sedentary lifestyle makes you put on weight and is not good for your health.

Cystitis and Candida

Two major problems that are on the increase amongst women and are both linked to toxicity are cystitis and candida. Cystitis is a bladder infection and it can be very uncomfortable with the sensation of burning in the urinary tract and the constant need to pass urine. It is thought that taking antibiotics may increase cystitis and vaginal thrush. Cystitis occurs when there are too many acids in the urinary tract, which may be caused by eating too much sugar, (bacteria thrive on sugar) also the over consumption of tea, coffee, alcohol and smoking which are also very acidic.

To combat cystitis, drink lots of boiled water, hot water is best for a cleansing effect and lots of cranberry juice. Cut out all acid forming foods, this includes meat, tea, coffee, alcohol, all sugars, orange juice, vinegar, cheese and spicy foods and eat lots of bland foods such as vegetables and especially celery, which is good for acidity and basmati rice. If you have ever had cystitis, then it is recommended to do a kidney cleanse and to increase the amount of water that you drink.

Candida Albicans is a yeast overgrowth, which is now reaching epidemic levels in women and is associated with many uncomfortable symptoms including irritability, depression, inability to concentrate, extreme fatigue, premenstrual tension, allergies, migraine, cystitis, acne and many other symptoms. Candida is on the increase because of the over consumption of sugar, stress, high levels of toxicity, antibiotics (which are also found in milk and meat) and mercury toxicity from amalgam fillings.

One of the difficulties with candida is that it is impossible to test accurately as to whether there is just a normal amount in the body or an overgrowth. In blood tests and faecal tests there are so many false negatives, whereas Kinesiology seems to give clearer answers, several doctors I have worked with agree on this. In Kinesiology we ask the body whether candida is present and whether there is an overgrowth and if so in which area and then one by one we test, which foods need to be cut out. Candidiasis is serious and people can die from it.

Some researchers believe that all people with immune compromised conditions including HIV/AIDS have candida infections. Some cancer experts have also said that they believe cancer starts with a yeast overgrowth, which increases toxic waste and then the cells start to malfunction. Candida is certainly a major and often unrecognised factor at the root of many diseases. Treating candida is not easy because it is very stubborn. Three steps need to be taken to combat candida. The immune system must be strengthened, the candida must be starved and friendly bacteria introduced into the intestinal tract. Antibiotics destroy the friendly bacteria and make the situation worse.

The best herb to take to strengthen the immune system is Lapacho, also known as pau d'arco. It can be taken both in capsule form and as a tea, ideally you should take both for a period of at least six months. You can take 4 - 6 capsules a day and drink up to six cups of lapacho tea. Lactobacillus acidophilus is most often given to repopulate the intestines with friendly bacteria or you can take live, fresh yogurt with meals, two to three times a day. Don't eat strained yogurt, you need both the curds and whey. Avoid fruit yogurts. Acidophilus does not agree with everyone and can cause diarrhoea. It is important to clean the colon and kidneys, as it is not so easy for the candida to take hold in a clean gut. Then healthy bacteria can be implanted through colon reflorastation.

Aloe Vera juice is recommended for its amazing healing qualities and antifungal action that can be helpful in treating candida. It is also full of essential minerals. Some Aloe Vera juice contains fructose, which is used as a natural sweetener and preservative, so it is best to test whether or not you can tolerate it to be sure. Black walnut tincture is also antifungal. Garlic, olive oil and turmeric are antimicrobial and can be taken with food. Tea tree oil is anti fungal and can be used as a mouthwash or douche.

Starving the candida means that you have to cut out everything that feeds it, this means a very strict diet. You have to cut out all sugar; candida thrives on sugar rich food including alcohol, soft drinks, fruit juices, dried fruits, fresh fruit, honey and molasses. Look for hidden sugars, for example in breakfast cereals, muesli and milk. Sugar is also in tinned, frozen, packaged and processed food. You also have to avoid all yeast promoting foods including bread, cakes, biscuits, crackers, self raising flour, mushrooms, soya sauce, stock cubes, cheese, nuts and fermented foods, spreads, marmite, vinegar, pickles and salad dressings. This means your main diet must be based mainly upon salads, vegetables, rice and oats.

It can take from 3 – 9 months to clear candida, depending on the severity of the problem. You need to be very strict about your diet for it to clear. After three months, if your symptoms have improved, you can begin to reintroduce foods slowly. You can begin with apples and cottage cheese and slowly other fruits and see the effect. (Avoid grapes and melons because of their high sugar content.) Avoid multi vitamins and selenium supplements, which are yeast sources. There is a question around apple cider vinegar; some people say it is helpful, others say no, you have to test if it is okay for you. Whilst on an anti candida diet, eat oatmeal porridge made with water or soya milk with a little added cinnamon once a day. Oats are nourishing and balancing for the intestines as well as providing bulk. Also drink herbal teas such quebra pedra for cleaning the kidneys, camomile, lapacho and green tea.

The anti candida diet takes patience and perseverance. Keep boosting the immune system by taking lapacho and detox the kidneys and liver, liver health is very important whilst clearing candida. Get lots of early sleep and rest, which is essential whilst the body is detoxifying. Stress is a major factor in candida and one of the causes, so try to keep stress to a minimum. It takes from 7 –10 days for the candida to start dying off and as the yeast dies off, there may be discomfort and cravings for sugar as the blood sugar level fluctuates.

4 – REJUVENATION

For thousands of years people have been searching for a magic elixir or formula that will rejuvenate and prevent the ageing process. The possibility of total rejuvenation is written in some of the ancient texts such as the Caraka Samhita. Some of the greatest Indian sages and Tibetans are said to have profound knowledge of how to prolong life, promote perfect health and youthfulness. Continuous streams of spiritual seekers flock to the East, hoping to learn the secrets of consciousness, eternal youth, perfect health and immortality. Throughout the years many great Yogis have been drawn to remote regions of the Himalayas and Tibet to explore and gain deeper knowledge on these subjects. There are said to be Tibetans who are hundreds of years old.

We know that the body has a great capacity for rejuvenation if given the right circumstances. What needs to be investigated is what will encourage and promote regeneration, rejuvenation and healing. We need a multifaceted approach, which includes as many things as possible to enable us to live a really healthy and fulfilling life.

Although our genes and hereditary factors have an influence on the aging process, we can extend our lifespan considerably by leading a more supportive lifestyle and having a positive mental attitude. Youthfulness is an internal state that is fuelled by an active spirit that is young at heart and has a passion for life. Many factors contribute to the acceleration or slowing down of the aging process. Inner peace, joy and fulfilment in life, play a major and crucial part in regeneration. A stress free attitude helps us maintain harmony and balance, and affects how we feel and everything we do. Spiritual practices including the regular practice of meditation can support and nourish us on a deep level. Through meditation, our intuition develops to a much higher degree and our senses become more refined and this enables us to make better choices.

In order for rejuvenation to occur, the body must be able to detoxify efficiently as well as being able to do the necessary repair and regeneration work. Detoxification removes toxins, acids and waste products from the body and improves the quality of the blood, the functioning of the organs and the assimilation of nutrients. Feeding the cells with life force energy and vital nutrients, which are obtained from pure foods is needed for sustenance and tissue repair. The full benefits of any rejuvenation programme will be minimalised without detoxification. By following many of the principles and suggestions given, you can regenerate and greatly improve your health. Everything depends upon your ability and willingness to adopt a more life enhancing and life supporting lifestyle.

By eating the right amount of good nourishing food and drinking lots of fresh water, implementing the principles of conscious eating, getting enough fresh air, life force energy and sunlight, we can nourish and support ourselves in the way that is needed. Add to that a good daily routine, enough rest, relaxation, good quality sleep and learning how to manage stress in the right way, moves us in the right direction towards radiant health.

Cellular Rejuvenation

The quality of your health and your life literally depend upon the health and vibratory level of your cells. The mind has an effect upon every part of the body, including each individual cell. How you feel will directly affect the health of your cells. If you are happy, you will have happy cells, if you are depressed, you will have depressed cells, if you constantly live in fear, you will have fearful cells. Unhappy, depressed or fearful cells become weak and lethargic and jeopardise the immune system. When you have joyful and blissful thoughts, the vibrational rate of the cells is higher and this promotes healing.

For regeneration of the cells to occur, they need proper nourishment. Incorrect eating habits, over indulgence, smoking, alcohol, lack of exercise, poor quality sleep, stress, and a lack of happiness and fulfilment in life cause degeneration and inhibit the absorption of vitamins and minerals. When the cells are properly cleansed and nourished, the aging process takes its natural pace, and the mind and body can remain vital and alert at any age.

Everything we ingest has an effect on the body, it can be nourishing and revitalizing or it can be clogging, depleting, poisoning and dehydrating. If you constantly eat dead food, you will be low in energy, the immune system will become weak and your metabolism will not function efficiently. Dead foods are those that do not have any life force energy, they include packaged, processed, tinned, frozen, microwaved food and leftovers. Nutritional deficiencies result from a lack of nourishing food and this causes premature degeneration. By selecting natural, high quality food including those from the superfoods list and by adding certain food supplements to your diet, you will nourish both your mind and all the cells of your body.

Old and decayed cells are constantly broken down and replaced by new cells but the quality of new cells depends upon the nourishment they receive and the environment they exist in. The quality of the blood and cellular vitality are dependent upon receiving enough vitamins, minerals and enzymes from pure, natural sources not from chemical man made sources. Oxygen is an important nutrient, which influences the lifespan and vitality of the cells. When the cells do not receive enough oxygen, they cannot regenerate properly. Both stress and smoking interfere with the breathing process and therefore seriously damage the cells, this can cause mutations and the cells can become cancerous. Releasing stress that has accumulated in the cells or in any other part of the body is an essential part of any rejuvenation programme. Specific breathing techniques such as pranayama or pranic breathing increase cellular purification and nourish the cells.

For optimum cell function and for rejuvenation to take place, accumulated wastes from the cells and the tissues must be eliminated on an ongoing basis. Degeneration occurs when there is more toxic waste than the body can efficiently eliminate. As we become older, our metabolism, assimilation and glandular activity slow down and metabolic wastes and fluids are not excreted at the same rate. How fast the body can repair or replace old cells and tissues indicates the level of health. When we aren't eliminating toxins and waste products at a fast enough rate, there will be a build up leading to an overload, which causes congestion, decay and disease. We can improve our metabolism by maximising the elimination of wastes from the body and by increasing our energy level through energy work.

To create a new, healthier body we can reprogramme the mind with uplifting thoughts of youthfulness, regeneration and vitality. We can visualize our cells being cleansed and renewed through the power of the mind but we also have to combine it with purification, oxygenation of the cells and proper nutrition. Repatterning changes the way we think. We can open closed neurological pathways in the brain and create new ones and restructure the cellular memory to bring about transformation.

Brain Power

The brain is the most important part of the nervous system, it controls every gland and organ in the body and sends messages to every part of the body via the spinal cord, and so it is vital to maintain optimal brain function. The brain needs to be constantly nourished with a good supply of well-oxygenated blood, which depends upon the absorption of vital nutrients from the food. Oxygen is the most important nutrient for the brain. Smoking deprives the brain of oxygen and kills brain cells. The effects of smoking can stay in the body for many years.

Yoga asanas, pranayamas (breathing techniques) and meditation increase the flow of energy throughout the whole body and help activate the different parts of the brain including the pineal and pituitary glands. It is said that we use only 5%-10% of our brain potential, imagine what we could achieve if we used our full brain potential. Although all Yoga asanas help rejuvenate the body, there are two asanas, which are said to specifically activate the different parts of the brain including the frontal lobes, the mid brain and the medulla at the back of the head. These two asanas are the shoulderstand and the headstand and they should be practised every day. However, they are advanced postures and before attempting them, the body needs to be prepared by other asanas, which help improve flexibility and energy flow. For those who are unable to do the full headstand, the preparation to the headstand is almost as effective. To receive the maximum effect, these two asanas should be practised in conjunction with pranayama and meditation.

Alternative nostril breathing is an excellent pranayama technique, which is known to activate the pineal and pituitary glands and to promote left and right brain co-ordination and improve memory and concentration. It can be practised before meditation or before sleep and the deeply relaxing effects will help improve the quality of your sleep. Regular massage of the neck and scalp with sesame oil, release tension and increase the circulation of blood to the different parts of the brain. There are many pressure points on the head, which can be worked to stimulate brain function.

When the mind and body are in a total state of peace and harmony and there is balance between the different systems of the body, then a natural, hormonal type substance called ojas can be released from the brain. Ojas has been called the nectar of the Gods or in modern day terms a bliss hormone. When ojas is activated in the brain, it flows down into the heart and it creates the experience of pure bliss. Ojas is considered to be the most sattvic substance and it nourishes all seven levels of the tissues. When ojas is present, there is a high level of vitality and it has the restorative power to change the physiology. Ojas increases when a sattvic state of mind dominates. A sattvic mind is calm, clear, illumined and alert and has the ability to be one pointed and focused with a good attention span. A rajasic mind is overactive, tense and easily irritated and has difficulty in concentrating. A tamasic mind is dull and lazy and has a low level of concentration, awareness or alertness. Meditation helps the mind to develop more sattvic qualities.

To keep the brain functioning well, we need a variety of mental stimulation and to develop both sides of the brain. The left side of the brain governs the intellectual and practical aspects and the right side governs the creative and intuitive aspects. Developing our full brain potential is possible through the expansion of consciousness, a refinement of the senses, sharpening our intuition and feeding the brain in the right way.

There are specific food substances, which improve brain functioning. Yogis consider ghee to be the most sattvic of all foods, it is nourishing for the brain and soothing for the nervous system. Ghee can be added to all foods and used in cooking. For those who drink milk, having a cup of warm milk before sleeping, with a teaspoon of ghee and a teaspoon of honey, with a pinch of cinnamon, cardamom and liquorice can improve the quality of your sleep. It is recommended to take about two teaspoons of ghee everyday. Also putting a little ghee into both nostrils and sniffing it up, lubricates the sinuses and the brain.

Chlorella and Lecithin are both considered to be important brain foods. Chlorella is an algae that improves brain function. Lecithin feeds the brain tissues and is an important source of choline, which protects the cells and nerve endings and helps with the breakdown of fats. It is available in granules and can be sprinkled on cereals, salads or cooked food. It comes from a natural source of soya.

There are two particular herbs that have an enlivening and restorative effect on the brain; these are guarana and ginkgo biloba. Guarana is a natural energizer from the Amazon and is one of the most popular herbs today. Guarana is a tonic and energy booster that eliminates mental and physical fatigue and has a stimulating effect on the brain and improves alertness and concentration. It is helpful for stress, anxiety, depression, migraine, headaches and pain. It can be taken on going or whenever you need it. Make sure to take pure guarana seed such as Rio guarana and not herbal combinations or extracts that contain guarana, as these do not produce the same effect.

87

Ginkgo biloba improves circulation to the extremities of the body and to the brain by dilating the blood vessels and increasing blood flow, whilst at the same time thinning the blood, making it less likely to clot. Gingko is known to improve memory and concentration and to stimulate overall brain function and has an antioxidant effect that protects nerve cells in the brain from deterioration. It needs to be taken for a period of time to see its effects. It is a very good remedy for menopausal women who experience symptoms of fogginess and dullness in the brain or lack of concentration, symptoms that are often associated with menopause. Research is currently being conducted into the effects of ginkgo in regards to Parkinson's and Alzheimer's disease. Gotu kola is an Indian herb, which is known to nourish and balance both sides of the brain and to activate the crown chakra.

It is important to take antioxidants to maintain the health of the brain. Amrit Kalash, Co-enzyme Q10 and Lapacho are three important antioxidants. Zinc and the B vitamins are also essential for brain function. Zinc and B6 are both found in bee pollen. Cinnamon, ginger and black pepper are antioxidants for the brain and can be included in cooking. Turmeric and black pepper help the brain absorb oxygen. Vitamin E improves the circulation to the brain. Magnesium is an important mineral for the brain and it also nourishes the bones and tissues. Beetroot contains a substance that stimulates brain function and basil and rosemary are two herbs that help increase mental alertness.

Protect your brain cells by avoiding smoky atmospheres and remember that smoking and alcohol cause degeneration of the brain cells.

Nourishing Every Level

For rejuvenation to take place, every part of us needs to be well nourished, the physical, the mental, the emotional and the spiritual. Lack of emotional nourishment can lead to addictions, compulsive behaviour and over indulgence. Nourishment comes in many forms, through sunlight, water, oxygen, food, sleep, rest and relaxation, life force energy, self-development and spiritual growth, fulfilling relationships, being in nature and whatever makes us feel truly good. By listening carefully to our deeper needs, we can learn how to nourish ourselves accordingly, we cannot expect others to do it for us, we have to do it for ourselves.

Even if you eat a nutritionally rich diet, it is still beneficial to take specific tonics, food supplements and herbs to strengthen and give an added boost to combat the stress and tension of everyday living and to aid in the regeneration and repair process. Stress and anxiety are ageing; they take their toll on the body and deplete nutrients. There are certain plants and substances called rasayanas and rejuvenatives, which have particular healing and restorative effects and are nourishing for the mind and body. Rejuvenative herbs help neutralize the damaging and degenerative effects of stressful living, it is recommended to take them after detoxification.

One of the most potent rejuvenatives is a highly concentrated Ayurvedic formula called Amrit Kalash, which has been described as an ambrosial nectar and is a potent, antioxidant. Amrit Kalash is a synergy of many precious herbs and fruits blended together according to an old traditional Indian recipe. It helps nourish, balance and strengthen the mind and the body. Many studies have evaluated its highly beneficial effects on the immune system and effectiveness against parasitic, fungal and bacterial infections. It enhances the body's recuperative and rejuvenative powers. Amrit is one of the main ingredients of Amrit Kalash and is described in the ancient Ayurvedic texts as the most beneficial of hundreds of herbal preparations. It works on the most refined, intelligent levels of the body and is said to help one attain longevity, strengthen the mind and body and improve memory and intelligence. It also decreases tumour formation.

Noni is a medicinal, healing fruit that grows in tropical areas such as the Polynesian islands and Hawaii. It is said to have remarkable healing powers and has been used for over two thousand years to heal many diseases in Polynesia, India and China. Noni is usually taken as a juice and today most of it is exported from Tahiti and Hawaii. Its curative qualities enhance the body's own healing abilities. It creates homeostasis through a balancing effect, which can normalize blood pressure (whether high or low) and blood sugar levels. It is said to relieve many ailments including inhibiting the growth of tumours and malignant cells. Noni is unique in its ability to regulate cellular function and to increase cellular regeneration of damaged cells. It contains multiple phytonutrients that feed the cells and acts as an adaptogen to normalise abnormal cell function. For this reason, it is valuable both as a rejuvenative and for healing many ailments. A lot of research has been done by doctors on the positive effects of Noni on cancer, tumours, arthritis, regulating blood pressure and sugar levels, allergies, inflammation, heart disease and others.

Another very interesting aspect about Noni is that it stimulates the pineal gland and increases the production of melatonin and serotonin. This has a regulating effect on sleep, mood and ovarian cycles and helps normalize and balance glandular function. Both the pineal gland and the thymus gland are known to shrink and become less active as we get older. Research shows that people with degenerative diseases have an under active thymus gland and it is suspected that low thymus function may be a major factor in many diseases. The thymus plays an important part in regeneration. Tapping the thymus gland, which is situated 4-5 cms below the collarbone and behind the sternum, increases immune action. Noni helps enliven the functioning of these two glands and has a normalizing effect on all the other glands. Adding Tahitian Noni to your daily diet as a regular food supplement and rejuvenative can greatly improve your health and help heal many ailments.

Bee products are superfoods, which are full of nutritional value. The bees give us the bountiful gifts of honey, pollen, propolis, royal jelly and beeswax. Honey is a vital food, rich in fructose and a natural source of energy. Honey is a wonderful alternative to sugar. We need to include the sweet taste in our diet and honey helps satisfy sweet cravings. Honey is a natural stimulant for the heart. Select the best quality 100% natural honey you can find but don't cook with honey as this creates a chemical change in the honey, which makes it lose its potency and medicinal qualities. If you add honey to herbal tea, wait for the tea to cool down before adding honey.

Bee pollen has remarkable qualities. It is a complete, wholesome food, containing, all the vitamins (high in B6), minerals and amino acids and is a rich source of protein. Bee pollen is a body builder and a potent tonic; it gives strength and stimulates all the functions of the body. It especially helps balance the metabolism, which is useful in glandular and weight problems. It is a natural antibiotic and controls bacteria in the intestines. It is helpful for diabetes, hypoglycaemia and arthritis. Bee pollen is non allergenic and relieves allergies that are airborne such as hay fever. It is high in zinc, which is good for the brain. If you suffer from allergies, it is helpful to start taking bee pollen at least three months before spring or autumn.

Royal Jelly is the superfood of the bees and reserved only for the Queen bee. It is full of all the vitamins and is rich in B vitamins, minerals, protein and amino acids. It enhances the body's metabolism and is an important supplement because it contains silicon, which aids cellular rejuvenation and benefits and improves skin texture.

Bee propolis is a sticky resin excreted from the trees. It is a natural food supplement with antibiotic properties. It is antibacterial, antiviral and antiparasitic and beneficial for inner wounds and inflammation. Bee propolis is valuable because it increases the rate of metabolism of the thymus gland and thereby stimulates the whole immunological system.

Co-enzyme Q10 is a vitamin like substance that is found in nearly all the cells of the body. It is considered to be the energy spark in the centre of the cell, which declines with age. It is recommended to take Co-enzyme Q10 to improve the health of the cells, tissues and organs. It helps slow down the aging process by fighting free radicals, which damage the cells and cause degeneration. Decades of research have found it to be effective in cardiovascular health. Many doctors now recommend it because of its ability to improve heart function and to prevent heart disease through the slowing down of the effects of cholesterol.

A special nourishing Ayurvedic recipe for feeding the deepest level of the tissues is made with ground almonds, which are good for the brain. Boil the almonds and remove the skin, which contains a poisonous substance, grind them and mix them with a teaspoon of honey and a teaspoon of ghee and a pinch of cinnamon and liquorice powder mixed with a little warm milk or water or rosewater. It becomes a paste and is delicious. It can be taken every day and is recommended after lovemaking, both for women and men as it feeds shukra, the reproductive tissue.

The body needs a strong immune system to build up strength and support all the functions of the body including fighting infections. When the immune system is weak, it becomes more vulnerable to the daily stresses of life. You are born with a certain level of immunity, which depends upon your basic constitution and hereditary factors and also whether you were breastfed. The breast milk of the mother is known to contain certain substances that improve immune functioning. Breast fed babies contract less childhood diseases due to having developed a stronger immune system. There is another type of immunity, which is known as fluctuating immunity, which is influenced by lifestyle, diet, stress, change of season and other factors since childhood. If your immunity is already low or compromised, you need to take extra care and more time to rest, relax, sleep and nurture yourself well. People who catch colds or flu every winter have a low immune response.

We must protect the body against free radicals, which damage the body's defence system and the cells, capillaries, veins, arteries and the heart. Free radicals destroy healthy cells and speed up the ageing process. They also attack the collagen, which holds together bone, cartilage and connective tissues. They can cause mutation of the cells, which can lead to cancer. Free radicals have been linked to degenerative diseases and are a major factor in premature aging. They are generated by stress and toxic chemicals found in the air, water and food and from smoking, alcohol, x-rays and over exposure to the sun. Antioxidants are substances, which scavenge free radicals and protect the body. They also fight allergens by strengthening the immune response.

Natural sources of antioxidants are found in fresh fruit and vegetables, especially grapes, oranges, yellow fruits, fresh carrot juice, spinach, broccoli, red pepper, parsley, sage, rosemary and green tea. To boost the immune system, we must feed the body well with a healthy, nourishing diet and keep alcohol to a minimum.

Lapacho (also known as Pao d'arco) is one of the best herbs to support immune functioning. It comes from Brazil, from the bark of a tree. It is used to strengthen and balance the immune system and is a powerful tonic containing a large amount of iron. It protects against free radicals and aids the spleen. The spleen is the largest organ of the lymphatic system; in Chinese medicine it is also regarded as a major energy centre. The spleen produces white blood cells and antibodies, which eliminate bacteria and help fight infections and destroys and removes old red blood cells.

It is recommended to take Lapacho whenever you feel unwell, physically low or tired, prone to colds or when your immune system needs an extra boost, also after taking antibiotics or other medicines. Children can drink Lapacho tea, which prevents them from getting colds and viruses. Research has been done on Lapacho in Brazil on immune system related diseases. In the hospitals they give Lapacho to cancer patients and have very good results. Gandhi was reputed to have drunk a cup of Lapacho tea every day and attributed it to his good health.

Echinacea is another well-known immune strengthening herb, but it has the disadvantage of its potency being reduced after about ten days. So it can only be taken for short periods of time, whereas Lapacho can be taken on going especially throughout the winter months.

Blood building foods improve immune functioning and the quality of the blood can be improved by eating foods, which are rich in chlorophyll such as green leafy vegetables, beetroot, seaweed, nettles, apricots, parsley and algae. Liquorice root enhances immune function and has anti tumour properties. Increase your daily intake of green foods and include broccoli, dandelion, parsley, coriander, green peppers, spinach, alfalfa and other dark green leafy vegetables both raw and cooked. Drink a daily green drink (use all the stalks and leaves that you cut off from the vegetables) and take a green supplement. Green foods are power foods, they increase energy, are natural antioxidants, immune enhancers and rich in enzymes.

Chlorella is one of the best green supplements known. It has been called the Jewel of the Far East. Millions of people in Japan take Chlorella where it is well known for its antioxidant properties. Chlorella is a sun powered super rich green algae. It is a wholefood not an extract and contains more chlorophyll than any other algae. It is one of the most scientifically studied foods; it is high in vitamins and contains 60% protein, (which makes it an essential food for vegetarians) 18 different amino acids and is rich in minerals especially iron, calcium, magnesium and phosphorus. It is one of nature's most powerful detoxifiers. Besides its cleansing effect on the bowels, liver and kidneys, it is active in cellular repair and promotes cellular reproduction by increasing haemoglobin. It can heal damaged tissues. With the depletion of minerals in the soil due to over cultivation and the use of pesticides and fertilizers, it is very important to take enough minerals. Minerals and trace elements improve metabolic functioning, aid hormone production and build strong bones. Minerals are best attained through natural sources, (unless there is a serious depletion), such as eating enough green foods and including aloe vera juice, chlorella and kelp in your diet. Chlorella also helps the body to produce interferon, which fights cancer and immune related diseases.

We have to take care of our heart, both on a physical and emotional level. On a physical level, we have to keep the blood as pure as possible through regular detoxification and taking antioxidants and by improving the circulation of the blood to the heart. Good circulation speeds up the healing process, removes toxins and wastes more efficiently and transports more vital nutrients to the cells. It is well known that eating a nutrient rich, vegetarian diet with only small amounts of animal protein is good for the heart. Research shows that diets which are high in animal protein, meat and dairy products, cause premature aging by clogging the arteries and the brain. Regular exercise, breathing exercises and reflexology, improve blood circulation to the heart. To maintain the elasticity of the arteries, we need silicon, which is needed to make collagen. The best sources of silicon are alfalfa, pollen and seaweed. Turmeric is a blood cleanser and circulatory tonic. The spices, cinnamon, cardamom, cayenne pepper and ginger are also heart tonics and can be used regularly. Garlic is good for the heart and circulation, also onions, leeks, carrots, oats, barley and olive oil.

Obviously you cannot take all of these supplements and rejuvenatives at once, you have to select according to your needs and to what is appropriate at a particular time. It is good to also alternate your supplements; this gives an extra boost when you start again. Kinesiology is the best tool to check which rejuvenatives, food supplements or herbs should be taken at any given time. (I teach a simple Kinesiology self check system in my Self Healing Seminar.)

Yoga

Yoga is one of my passions and I have been teaching it for many years. It offers a never-ending exciting exploration into life. Yoga is a way of being; it is a process of awakening that can lead to enlightenment. It is a rejuvenation system in itself. Although Yoga originated in India, people of all religions practise Yoga all over the world. The true purpose of Yoga is union, a harmonious integration of body, mind, spirit and soul. Yoga prepares the student for the experience of self-realization and self-actualisation through releasing the blocks, which prevent this from happening. Yoga opens the doors of perception and introduces you to the deeper realities of life. By expanding consciousness and clearing the illusions and the superficial, it gives one the ability to discover the deeper meaning of life.

There are many different systems of Yoga and probably the most well known is Hatha Yoga, which prepares the body for transformation and the development of higher states of consciousness. Through cultivating a deeper awareness of the connection between the body, the mind and the senses and between the inner and the outer, we can progress to more expansive levels of being. If the physical body is blocked, then the energy system will be blocked too and the other way round. We need to release energy blocks so that the kundalini energy, the powerful life force in the body can awaken. Yoga helps develop an ongoing state of awareness that influences everything we do, including how we breathe, stand, speak, eat and act.

Other popular systems of Yoga are Kriya Hatha Yoga, Ashtanga Yoga, Iyengar Yoga and Kundalini Yoga. For the purpose of this book, I will focus on the aspects of Yoga, which relate to improving your health. By regularly practising asanas (yogic physical postures) you can increase your energy level and improve flexibility. I love teaching Yoga, both private and individual classes and learn something from every class I teach. It is wonderful to see the changes in people after they practise Yoga for a period of time. The beauty of Yoga is that you can practise it at any age and continue to do so for the rest of your life. Some of the greatest Yoga teachers are in their nineties and even older and are an absolute inspiration, their vitality flows abundantly, they enjoy radiant health and their minds are crystal clear.

Even if you lead a very busy life, try to make time for at least fifteen minutes of asanas in the morning and another fifteen minutes in the evening, then you will start to see many changes in the way you look and feel. I recommend doing the Sun Salutation and a few standing postures in the morning and sitting and lying postures in the evening. For this purpose, I created two Yoga videos, Yoga for Health for people who either cannot get to a class or want to do more practise at home and Yoga for Pregnancy. If you can, try to attend at least one

Yoga class a week to learn more about breathing, energywork, relaxation, meditation and more advanced postures.

If you are pregnant, it is very beneficial to practise Yoga and it will help prepare you for the birth. Please check first with your doctor to make sure you do not have any complications with your pregnancy and that it is all right for you to practise Yoga. Generally speaking, if you have been exercising regularly and feel well, it is okay to start Yoga at any time, if however, you have not exercised for a long time or are not fit, your doctor may advise you to wait until after the first three months of pregnancy especially if this is your first baby. It is also recommended to wait for at least forty days after giving birth before resuming your Yoga practise.

There are many different ways of teaching Yoga and classes vary according to the specific tradition of the teacher. Although the basic asanas are the same, there are thousands of variations to choose from. Most people begin with Hatha Yoga and enjoy it as a good exercise routine, however Yoga offers much more. As the student progresses and becomes more aware of the bodymind connection and more health conscious, they may wish to go onto other aspects of Yoga such as learning about the energy system, healing and further self-development.

Yoga works on many different levels at the same time. It improves posture, stamina and strength and releases tightness and tension. It helps the internal organs by increasing the elimination of toxins and acids and improves the functioning of the spine, the muscles and glands and increases the circulation of the blood and lymph flow. As the breathing capacity improves, the heart and lungs are also strengthened. Yoga is very beneficial for women because of the balancing effects on the nervous system and endocrine system and the more subtle level of the body, the energy system. By becoming more aware and learning to relax, you calm the mind, dissolve stress and balance the hormones. As the vital energy flow increases, it purifies the energy channels called nadis.

Your body is a perfect mirror. It reflects both your strengths and your weaknesses and shows up what needs attention. In Yoga we work from the spine, a lot of attention is paid to the spine. It is said that you are as young or old as your spine; no other exercise gives as much attention to the spine. Thousands of nerves are attached to the spine and extend outwards to every organ of the body. All of these nerves are stimulated whilst doing asanas. Loss of spinal flexibility causes vertebrae to contract and press on the nerves, this restricts the proper functioning of the organs and glands and causes problems. To maintain youthfulness, the spine must remain flexible.

Yoga works to revitalize the mind and body by clearing blocks and promoting regeneration. Mastery of the mind and body are taught in order to set the spirit free. When you learn how to calm the restless fluctuations of the mind and to develop one pointed concentration, you will find that helps every area of your life.

Inner Beauty, Outer Beauty

True beauty is a radiance that is attractive and does not diminish with age. Inner peace, harmony and balance are essential components of any natural beauty regime and can help activate the bliss hormone, ojas. Beautiful skin comes from radiant health. Your skin is a mirror of what is happening inside your body. Stress, imbalanced eating habits and a build up of toxic wastes, trigger and aggravate skin problems and allergies. In order to cure these conditions permanently, you have to detoxify regularly, make the necessary dietary changes and pay attention to your stress level and emotional health.

A skin care routine should be geared towards cleansing, exfoliation, protection and nourishment. The skin absorbs whatever is put on it and transmits it into the bloodstream. Many beauty products contain a high percentage of harsh chemicals, preservatives and alcohol. The beauty industry is big business and millions of pounds are spent in making attractive packaging and on clever advertising but most of the products do not live up to what they promise. Select products, which are as natural as possible and use natural preservatives. Rosewater is a wonderful tonic for the face. Ghee and sesame oil are natural beauty products for the skin. Essential oils are very useful for nourishing and regenerating the skin. (More on essential oils in Chapter 5 - Nature's Gifts).

For good skin you have to pay attention to your diet and regularly detoxify your kidneys and liver. Orange foods are rich in vitamin A, which is needed for healthy skin. Orange juice is beneficial but don't drink too much of it as excess can cause acidity. Drink a glass of carrot juice every day for your skin and eat dried, soaked apricots. Sesame, pumpkin and sunflower seeds are rich in zinc, which is necessary for the repair work of the skin. Avocado is high in vitamins A and E and you can combine avocado and honey for a facemask. Lemon juice can be used as an astringent for greasy skin. Clay masks are the best for deep cleansing and Dead Sea products are very helpful for people with serious skin problems. I have also found Noni juice improves the skin because of its cellular detoxification properties.

Most hair products contain large amounts of chemicals. Choose companies that specialize in natural shampoos and conditioners that are plant based. If you colour your hair, ask for vegetable dyes or highlight the hair instead. If the dye and bleach go into the pores of the scalp to the brain, this can be harmful and cause blood poisoning.

Ayurveda recommends regular oleation of the skin through sesame oil massage as a part of your daily routine. Asian women tend to have very good skin; they know the secret of using ghee and sesame oil and how to take care of their skin without paying a lot of money. They add ghee to everything they cook and even put it on their face; ghee is considered to be the ultimate nourishment for the skin. Don't buy readymade ghee unless you are sure it is fresh and from a very good source. It should be bright yellow in colour.

Abhyanga, daily sesame oil massage is considered an essential part of any rejuvenation treatment in all Ayurvedic clinics. It is followed by a herbal steam bath. It only takes a couple of minutes every morning before your shower to gently massage the whole body with sesame oil. On weekends or when you have more time, you can leave the oil on longer. You don't need to use soap on the skin except for your private parts, the sesame oil does the work of detoxifying the skin and removing impurities. After the shower, gently pat the body dry. A thin film of oil will remain on the skin. You may also add essential oils to the sesame oil if you desire. It is recommended not to do massage during menstruation as the body is already eliminating more during this time, so instead you can massage just the feet. It is also very soothing to massage the head and ears regularly with sesame oil. There are many acupuncture points in the ears, massaging the ears triggers the ear reflexes and the ears start to get hot.

Sesame oil massage promotes youthfulness and lustre of the skin and balances the nervous system. Sesame oil is antibiotic, antifungal and antiflammatory and contains antioxidants, which retard the effects of ageing and can halt the growth of cancer cells. It penetrates the skin, which is the largest organ of elimination, draws out toxins and increases circulation. It also calms and nourishes the nerves and lubricates the seven layers of the tissues, the muscles and joints.

Make sure to buy cold pressed sesame oil, preferably organic, not the sesame oil, which is used for cooking. Sesame oil needs to be cured before using it by warming it gently. Add a few drops of water to the heated sesame oil (don't let it boil) and as soon as it starts to crackle, remove it from the heat and allow it to cool, then it is ready for use. In winter months, you can gently reheat the oil, for a warming, soothing effect.

Every woman deserves to have regular treatments that support and nourish her and help regenerate and relax her mind and body, Massage, aromatherapy, reflexology and healing are ways to give yourself extra care and attention, especially at times when you feel stressed or tired or before menstruation. This is a gift you can give to yourself and you should do it as often as you can.

In the following chapters, you will find many other ways to nourish and regenerate yourself physically, emotionally, energetically and spiritually.

5 – NATURE'S GIFTS

Herbs, Essential Oils and Flower Essences

Nature offers us an abundance of gifts in the form of sunlight, fresh air, water, food and herbs. Herbal remedies have been used for thousands of years and passed down from generation to generation. It is said that for every imbalance, health problem or disease there is a corresponding herb, plant or flower, which can heal or recreate balance. All roots and leaves have medicinal qualities but they must be taken in the correct dosage. Any herb, which grows plentifully is good for something. The expertise lies in selecting the right herbs for a person and their particular imbalances or disease. Everyone is different and responds differently, what works for one person may not work for another. Always trust your intuition and if something doesn't feel right or there is a strong reaction to any food, herb or essence don't take it.

There are 1000s of herbs to choose from and many wonderful books that give detailed information but for more serious complaints it is always good to consult with a herbalist. The following is an introduction to the most commonly used herbs, essential oils and flower essences, and specifically those I know well and have worked with for many years and recommend to my clients.

Herbs are very therapeutic and can be used in a variety of ways; they can be drunk as herbal teas, added to cooking or to salads. Herbs can be obtained fresh or dry and taken in the form of tinctures, tablets or in capsule form. Experiment carefully for herbs are powerful. If you are unsure, take less rather than more whilst you observe the effects on your body. Herbs are usually slow healers, so you need to take them over a period of time, most often a couple of months. You can also grow your own herbs so as to have fresh herbs available whenever you need them. Create a herb garden or grow herbs in pots on the windowsill. The most popular herbs to grow are lavender, mint, basil, rosemary, aloe vera, sage and thyme.

Many herbs have an antibiotic effect and can be used instead of chemically prepared antibiotics, which weaken the immune system and have unpleasant side effects. When herbs are combined, they have a synergistic effect, which can be more powerful. They also contain many vitamins and minerals, which are easy for the body to digest and assimilate. It is not enough however just enough to take supplements or herbs, you also have to pay attention to your diet and lifestyle. Remember if you add honey to herbal tea, wait for it to cool first.

Herbs have different effects, some are healing and restorative, others are tonics. Some are stimulants and improve circulation and open blocked channels or have a purging and cleansing effect that moves impurities out of the body. Diuretics increase the secretion of urine and stimulate the kidneys, astringents lessen excessive discharge and have a drying effect, and expectorants promote the expulsion of excess mucous. Nervines are natural antidepressants and tranquillisers, which stabilize the nervous system.

It is preferable to select herbs that are either grown in natural and unpolluted areas where the prana is high or herbs that are classified as organic. The herbs from the Amazon, Peru and the Himalayas are particularly potent because of the high amount of prana in these regions. I have worked with the Amazonian herbs for many years and find them very powerful; they have tremendous medicinal effects. Scientists and phytochemists are investigating the folklore of native medicines to discover more answers to our modern ailments. The mind and body need to be treated holistically and it must be remembered that all systems are linked and interactive but for the sake of basic understanding and as an introduction to the herbs, I have listed them according to the different systems of the body.

Herbs from the Amazon

One of the most valuable, therapeutic and widely used plants in the Amazon is guarana. Guarana is a natural energy plant. It is a tonic, a stimulant and an energy booster both physically and mentally. It is also one of the best natural remedies for migraines, headaches, depression, exhaustion, inertia and chronic fatigue. It is helpful when trying to give up addictions including coffee, tea, smoking or certain foods. Guarana contains tiny amounts of caffeine, which is slowly released into the bloodstream, it acts on the body in a totally different way to coffee, which gives an up and down effect on the nervous system and is addictive. Guarana is not addictive and can be taken on going for periods of time or just when you need it. It soothes the nervous system, so it is helpful for all stress related and anxiety symptoms and it increases stamina when feeling weak or recovering from illness. Whenever your energy feels low take guarana. It should be taken in the morning so as not to energize you in the evening and interfere with your sleep. It is also great when you are travelling or need to get over jet lag. Rio guarana is pure seed and the best source I have come across, it is available in capsule form.

Lapacho also known as pau d'arco is the first choice for the immune system. It is good to start taking it at the onset of winter as a preventative. It can be taken on going unlike Echinacea, which loses its potency effect after ten days. It is used in many hospitals in Brazil as a natural antibiotic and is helpful in fighting infections, colds, viruses, fungus, candida and parasites. It also stimulates new cell growth.

Quebra Pedra is a kidney tea from the Amazon, (previously mentioned in the detoxification chapter) which is helpful for cleaning the kidneys and the ureters and breaking down stones in the kidney, gall bladder and bladder. It is recommended as a general detoxifier.

A really important herb for women from the Amazon is Pfaffia, also known as Brazilian ginseng. This is one of the best tonics available for women; it is a natural hormone balancer and powerful nutritional supplement. It is considered to be one of the most effective natural alternatives to hormone replacement therapy. It is an adaptogen, which means it helps the body to produce, increase or decrease the amount of hormones that are secreted. If the body needs more oestrogen or progesterone it will help the body to produce it naturally and keep adapting according to the body's needs. Keeping the hormones in balance is absolutely essential for women. Chemically made hormones interfere with the body's natural intelligence whereas adaptogens encourage the body to produce the necessary hormones naturally. Pfaffia is helpful with the symptoms of menopause and premenstrual tension and emotional imbalance; it is also helpful for vaginal dryness during menopause.

The Amazonian Indians take Pfaffia for healing and for its rejuvenative powers of regenerating new cell growth. It is rich in phytoestrogens and is high in amino acids and trace minerals including iron, magnesium, potassium and zinc and vitamins A, B, and C. It is one of the best natural food supplements for women. Brazilian ginseng should not be confused with any other type of ginseng, which have a totally different effect and tend to be heating. Pfaffia is also said to inhibit the growth of tumours and prevent premenstrual tension. It is helpful in regulating menstruation and may improve fertility. It should not be taken by pregnant women or women on HRT. Pfaffia has been well researched in Russia and Japan and is being used around the world by doctors and in clinics to treat cancers and tumours related to the reproductive system.

Maca is a root, which comes from Peru where it is taken as a food supplement. It is rich in protein, vitamins and minerals and has a high content of alkaloids, which appear to stimulate the body's hormone system and increase fertility through its aphrodisiacal powers. It is helpful both for women and men, it increases sex drive and sperm count in men and increases libido. It is good to use after menopause where there is low libido. It is being compared as a natural alternative to viagra. It contains amino acids and is rich in magnesium and phosphorus.

Herbs for the Female Reproductive System

I have already mentioned pfaffia, Brazilian ginseng (from the Amazon). Other useful herbs are agnus castus, black cohash, damiana, wild yam, motherwort, evening primrose and sage. It is not recommended to take any female balancing herbs if you are pregnant or on hormone replacement therapy.

Agnus castus (also known as vitex or chasteberry) is a plant oestrogen and hormone balancer, which helps with the normal production of oestrogen and progesterone. It is particularly effective in regulating periods, which are irregular or too heavy or menstrual flooding where there is pain and uterine cramps during menstruation. It is prescribed also for uterine cysts. It can help with migraine headaches, which are brought on by hormonal imbalances and premenstrual tension. Black cohash brings on late periods and triggers labour. It contains estrogenic substances and helps with period pains and cramps and can be combined with agnus castus. It can be combined with pfaffia for hot flushes and night sweats when necessary.

Damiana is a herb used by the Mexican Indians. It has an exotic taste and makes a wonderful tea. It is an aphrodisiac and a tonic both for the reproductive system and for the nervous system and can be drunk regularly. It lifts your spirits and increases libido and is very helpful for menopausal women. Wild yam is generally taken for infertility and can increase sperm count in men. It is good for uterine pain and pain after childbirth and to increase milk production.

Motherwort is a very good herb and is most often taken as a tincture to counteract the emotional effects of reproductive and menstrual problems. It is a comfort herb and gives emotional support and is helpful during menstruation and menopause or where shock has affected the menstrual cycle. It also lowers the blood pressure. Evening primrose contains essential fatty acids and hormone like substances; it is usually taken as a nutritional substance or used as oil in massage. It is helpful for cystitis, bladder infections and cysts. Sage is rich in phytoestrogens and is helpful for hot flushes and night sweats. It should not be taken for long periods of time or if there is high blood pressure.

Herbs for the Nervous System

Many women suffer from stress, anxiety, restlessness, depression, insomnia or moodiness. The most common herbs for the nervous system are guarana, chamomile, lavender, lemon balm, orange blossom, rose, St. John's wort, valerian and passionflower. There are herbs, which sedate, soothe and calm and herbs, which uplift and support. Herbs from both groups can be combined according to one's needs.

Rio guarana is one of the best herbs for stress and depression. It is taken every day by millions of Brazilians as a tonic to energize and uplift and to combat stress and fatigue. Dr. Bach's rescue remedy flower essence is helpful in times of crisis or to calm you down when you are upset. If you can't relax because you have too many thoughts, you can take white chestnut flower essence, which calms the mental processes.

One of the most well known herbs for depression is St. John's wort. It has been called the prozac of the plant world and is used for mild to moderate depression. It is a safe herb when taken alone but it does not combine well with other prescription drugs especially blood thinning drugs or contraceptives. Women have become pregnant whilst taking the pill and St. John's wort at the same time. It should also not be taken whilst sunbathing, exposure to the sun whilst taking this herb can cause discolouration of the skin.

Chamomile and lemon balm (melissa) are soothing herbs and can be taken alone or together. They are both gentle herbs suitable for mild anxiety, tension and irritability, good for relaxing and unwinding at the end of a tiring day. Lemon balm is an elevating tonic for the nervous system and mind and is also good for circulation. Lime blossom is soothing and relaxing and reduces tension. Lavender is a wonderful herb with a multitude of uses. It is a relaxing and soothing herb and helpful for depression, headaches, pain and cramps. It can be taken alone or combined with any other herb.

Orange blossom is calming and good for headaches and indigestion caused by nervous tension. The wonderful neroli oil is distilled from the orange blossom. Hibiscus and rose petals are good for the heart and releasing the emotions where there is holding, tightness or grief. Passionflower, valerian and rosehips are helpful for sleeplessness. Passionflower is a mild sedative and useful for restlessness especially before menstruation or during menopause. Valerian is stronger and recommended for insomnia; it is also helpful when trying to break addictions. Avoid taking sleeping pills, which are addictive and depress brain function causing a zombie like state. This creates a never-ending cycle of needing stimulants like coffee to keep awake in the day, which irritate the nervous system and interfere with the natural sleep pattern and creates restlessness or lack of good quality sleep at night.

Basil is good for mental fatigue and depression and elevates the nervous system. Grow basil in pots in the kitchen and eat one or two leaves a day. Soothing herbal teas late in the evening enhance relaxation; choose from lavender, melissa (lemon balm) and passiflora (passion flower) and damiana. There are also special Ayurvedic teas and oils, to be used at night. If you have more serious sleep problems then you can try valerian and looking at the deeper cause of stress, which prevents you from sleeping.

Herbs for the Digestive System

The most popular herbs for the digestive system are aloe vera, dandelion, burdock root, sage, cloves, coriander and chaparrel. Aloe vera was already mentioned in detail in the detoxification chapter. It is one of the most valuable plants for healing all digestive disorders and for repairing the tissues. It can be drunk on a daily basis as a supplement and is one of the best natural remedies for constipation.

Dandelion is an excellent herb for detoxification and sluggish digestion and can be combined with burdock root as a herbal cleanse. It is rich in vitamins and minerals especially potassium. It is helpful in all liver and gall bladder disorders and prevents bloating during menstruation. Drink dandelion coffee as an alternative to coffee or chicory based drinks. Burdock root helps replenish lost minerals during detoxification and is also a blood purifier. Sage is a powerful herb, which stops putrefaction of the bowel. It increases peristaltic action in the intestines and gets things moving and is useful for diarrhea and anemia.

Coriander is the only natural substance, which efficiently clears heavy metal deposits from the body including mercury, lead and aluminium. It can also clear the body of amalgam, which may still be present in the body after amalgam fillings have been removed. It is thought that we all have toxic metals in our bodies and this can cause slow poisoning of the blood and liver, another reason to regularly detoxify your liver. Add a tablespoon of fresh coriander to your salad or food every day to clear out the metals. Many symptoms including depression and weakness and even Alzheimer's' are thought to be related to toxic metal poisoning.

Chaparrel is used by the Native Americans as a blood purifier and considered to be a healing plant for many diseases including cancer, viruses, herpes, digestive disorders, rheumatism and arthritis. It must be taken in small quantities otherwise it can be toxic.

Lavender kills bacteria and parasites and thyme is antiparasitic. Chamomile is soothing for a weak stomach. Parsley is good for digestion and is high in vitamins and minerals, Mint and peppermint are used mainly for digestive and intestinal disorders but also as an inhalant for chest disorders. Oregano stimulates the flow of bile and is helpful for intestinal problems. Milk thistle is a tonic for the liver and has a cleansing effect on the liver. It is useful in skin conditions including psoriasis.

Herbs for the Circulatory System

Gingko biloba is one of the most popular herbs today for enhancing circulation to the brain. It is called brain food because it increases the supply of blood, oxygen and nutrients to the brain and tissues and thereby improves brain function. It also helps improve memory and mental clarity and increases blood flow to the heart and the extremities, skin, eyes, inner ear and other vital organs and helps cramps in the legs. It is a very good herb to take during menopause if there is mental disorientation during hormonal changes. Many women have found enormous relief after taking Ginkgo and are able to work, concentrate and focus better. It needs to be taken regularly and it may take four to eight weeks to become really effective. Gingko can be combined with guarana for energy or with pfaffia the women's tonic. Gingko should not to be taken with blood thinning medicines. It is said to be useful in the early stages of Alzheimer's.

Where the circulation is sluggish use dandelion, sage or rosemary or combine them. For high blood pressure drink lemon balm and for low blood pressure drink dandelion or sage. Orange blossom is an antidepressant and good for anxiety and is a tonic for the heart.

Herbs for the Urinary System

Quebra pedra has already been mentioned as being one of the most useful herbs for the urinary system. There an important connection between the reproductive system and the urinary system, so the cleansing of the urinary system is essential in all reproductive disorders. Before I discovered quebra pedra I used to make my own kidney tea from 7 different herbs, which was effective but time consuming, now I use quebra pedra instead. Cystitis is very uncomfortable, for emergency treatment drink cranberry juice to relieve the discomfort and lots of hot boiled water to clear out the infection. Then drink quebra pedra for at least a month to clear the ureters.

Dandelion and parsley are helpful for fluid retention and oedema. Cleaver helps stimulate the lymph system. Juniper is cleansing and helpful in cystitis and arthritis. It promotes the elimination of uric acid. It is most often used as an essential oil, which is very strong and should be used sparingly. Nettle is an astringent, tonic, diuretic and blood cleanser.

Herbs for the Respiratory System

Sage is a tonic for the lungs and helpful in throat, gum and mouth infections. Oregano is useful for bronchitis. Lobelia is an old antidote to poison, but was also used for asthma and respiratory problems. Hyssop is helpful for asthma, coughs and colds. Basil and Rosemary can both be used for respiratory problems. Thyme is good for coughs and inflammation of the lungs. It is a strong antiseptic and decongestant, useful for chest infections such as bronchitis and asthma. It is an immune stimulant and helps produce white blood cells. Hyssop loosens phlegm and is helpful in asthma.

Other Herbs

There are many wonderful Ayurvedic herbs, spices and oils including those, which specifically balance each body type, vata, pitta and kapha. Vata tea, spice and oil, calm, sooth and balance the nervous system. Pitta works with the fire element and cools the fire in the body and heated emotions. Kapha stimulates and gets things going, it releases heaviness, sluggishness and stagnation.

Other herbs of interest are sideritis, roseox, gotu kola, ashwagandha, cat's claw, sarsparilla, black walnut and essaic. Sideritis is found mainly in Mediterranean countries and is a natural iron supplement. Roseox is a supplement, which has anti-oxidant properties that can rejuvenate the cells and tissues and prevent cancer. It can also eliminate heavy metals from the tissues. Gotu Kola is an Indian herb, which is known as food for the brain and is a memory enhancer; it balances both the right and left sides of the brain. It is also a tonic for purifying the blood and helpful against stress and anxiety. It is sometimes added to natural based facial creams as it enhances collagen synthesis Ashwagandha is an Ayurvedic rasayana, which helps with stress, ensures good sleep and is helpful for the heart. Cats claw from Peru is helpful for arthritis. Black walnut is usually taken as a tincture and is helpful to clear worms, ringworm, tapeworm, parasites and fungal infections.

Herbs during pregnancy

Be very careful of taking herbs during pregnancy as some are uterine stimulants and may have an adverse effect on the foetus. The following herbs are said to be safe during pregnancy, camomile, ginger, lemon balm, lavender and aloe vera. Camomile and ginger are both good for morning sickness. Lemon balm and lavender are safe calming and soothing herbs to use during pregnancy and to help relieve nausea. Aloe vera is good for constipation during pregnancy. Fennel (not to be taken during pregnancy) is good for breastfeeding mothers and promotes milk production and helps babies' colic. Sage reduces milk production when weaning. (Never take sage during pregnancy). Chamomile is also a good tea for colicky babies and restless children.

First aid treatment

For cuts or burns use Dr. Bach's Rescue Remedy cream. For bruises and sprains and the relief of pain, use Arnica ointment, which is antiseptic and anti-inflammatory, but it should not be used on cuts or broken skin.

Essential oils

The value and benefits of aromatic plants and essential oils have been known and appreciated by many cultures all over the world for centuries. Essential oils are extracted from flowers, citrus fruits, herbs, trees, and spices. Essential oils can be divided into different categories, regulators, which help balance, sedatives, which calm and stimulants and euphorics, which uplift and change your mood. There are also oils which are spiritually uplifting and whose effects are more subtle and are used in healing or meditation.

All essential oils can be used alone or blended with other oils to create a synergistic effect, which is more powerful. Blending is an art, finding the right combination of essential oils for a particular person and their specific needs at that time. For this reason many people prefer to buy oils, which are already blended. The most wonderful selection of blended oils, which I have come across and give to my clients are the Maharishi Ayurveda essential oil blends. Besides the traditional vata, pitta and kapha oils, there are oils for the mind, to calm the emotions, for vitality and strength, for bliss and joy, for times of transition (also recommended for menopause), to help menstruation, to improve breathing, for the joints and the muscles and oils for the night.

Essential oils are most often used in massage or in a burner. There is a profound difference in having a massage with essential oils or a massage with just a base oil. As well as the benefits of aromatherapy on the physical body, another interesting aspect is the effect of essential oils on the mind and the emotions and their ability to transform our psychological state. Essential oils have been used traditionally in temples and in rituals or in rites of passage. The power of essential oils should not be underestimated; they are a system of healing in their own right and they can be combined as an added benefit to enhance any system of healing.

Always buy the best and most expensive oils that you can, you literally get what you pay for. Cheap oils are a cheap imitation and will not have the same potency or result. Essential oils should be used sparsely; it is not a question of using more so as to have more benefit, in most cases a few drops are enough. Smell is very important in your selection of oils, if you don't like the smell of a particular oil or blend, don't use it, always trust your intuition, if you are drawn to a particular oil then it will most likely be the oil that you need.

Oils from different parts of the world can vary tremendously, for example there are many varieties of lavender and some are stronger or more potent than others. Essential oils have many attributes and uses and the following information is an introduction to some of the ways that essential oils can be used. For more serious complaints or imbalances please consult with a qualified aromatherapist.

Essential oils can be used in massage, in oil burners and vaporizers or added to the bath, sauna, or pot pourri. They can be used on a tissue or in bowls of water around the house or diluted as a perfume. Essential oils should not be used directly on the skin (with the exception of lavender) as they are highly concentrated but should be diluted in a base oil. On average, (some oils are stronger and so less is needed) dilute 5 drops of essential oil in 10mls of base oil, about one tablespoon. Don't keep oils in the bathroom, the humid environment is not good for them, neither should they be exposed to the sun. They are best kept in the dark, in a cupboard or drawer. Traditionally essential oils are stored in dark brown or dark blue glass bottles to preserve them.

The best base oil to use for massage is almond oil. For daily self-massage it is better to use sesame oil, which has detoxifying qualities, but for massage treatments, almond oil is lighter and easier to spread. A few drops of apricot kernel oil, avocado oil or wheatgerm oil can be added to the base oil for dry and dehydrated skins. Evening primrose oil can be added for problem skins and during menopause. Wheatgerm oil is sometimes added as a preservative but some people don't like the smell of it and it should be avoided if there is a wheat allergy. Jojoba can be added to the base oil for oily skin.

Women spend a fortune on buying expensive creams and products for their skin but essential oils can also be used to enhance and preserve the skin. They do not contain any harmful chemicals, preservatives or alcohol, which have a drying and damaging effect upon the skin. There are many beautiful older women with youthful looking skins who use only essential oils on their skin. Many natural facial products are based upon essential oils. Cleopatra was said to attribute her beautiful skin to a secret blend of essential oils.

Cellular rejuvenation is the key to a youthful skin. The two most important essential oils, which have a cytophylactic effect on the skin and stimulate new cell growth, are neroli and lavender. Palmarosa is also a cell regenerating oil. These can be mixed with any of the richer base oils such as peach kernel, avocado and wheatgerm. Geranium, jasmine, rose and frankincense are also good for older skins and carrot and frankincense are recommended for wrinkles.

Geranium and lavender have a balancing effect on the skin, whereas camomile, neroli and rose are soothing. Elemi has a restorative effect and can be added to speed up the healing process. Juniper is helpful in acne, psoriasis and eczema (use sparingly as it is a strong oil). Bergamot inhibits where there is bacterial infection and is good for acne and other infected skin conditions. Lavender is soothing where there is inflammation and myrrh is useful in the treatment of wounds and was used to treat soldiers' wounds during the war. Rosewood and Rosa mosqueta from the Andes help heal scar tissue. Tea tree is a natural antiseptic and can be dabbed on spots, bites and cuts.

The best oils for dry skin are neroli, rose, geranium, bergamot and frankincense, for normal skin geranium, lavender and jasmine and for oily skins bergamot, cypress and juniper. Maharishi Ayurveda has an excellent face oil, called Radiant Skin, which is a combination of seven pure essential oils. It can be used on its own or under your cream and as a treatment at night. Rosa mosqueta is a rich rose oil that comes from a beautiful wild rose that grows high in the Andes. All rose oil is good for the skin but this particular rose oil is highly beneficial in preventing premature ageing of the skin. It is one of the beauty secrets of Latin American women. Rosa mosqueta is high in essential fatty acids, which have regenerating effects on the skin. It is said to be richer than evening primrose oil or vitamin E. It also contains retinal, a precious skin nutrient that is related to vitamin A.

Many dermatologists recommend this oil because of its ability to heal scar tissue.

If you are new to working with essential oils, then I would suggest that you experiment slowly. Always use less rather than more and use just a couple of drops to see the effect. The most important essential oils to become familiar with and that are easy to use are lavender, tea tree, bergamot, geranium, rosemary, thyme and eucalyptus. These could be referred to as your basic needs kit.

Lavender is the most versatile of all oils and can be used for almost anything and it mixes well with all other oils. If you don't particularly like the smell of lavender you will find that when it is mixed with other oils it changes and enhances the other oils. Lavender can be used for any sort of pain including headaches, backaches and menstrual pain. It is the one oil, which can be applied directly onto the skin; it promotes healing and can be used on burns, sunburn and wounds, (for these it is better diluted). It is an antidepressant, antiseptic and very soothing. In a low dilution it is suitable for fretful babies. If you don't know which oil to use, then choose lavender. Lavender can be combined with chamomile, which is a very soothing oil and suitable for calming panic attacks. Always carry lavender and tea tree oil with you when you travel.

Tea tree is your basic first aid oil. Knowledge of tea tree oil comes from the Aborigines who use it for just about everything. It is not a pleasant smelling oil but it is a powerful antiseptic and immune stimulant. It is very strong, so you need only one or two drops. It is active against bacteria, fungi, viruses, warts, skin infections, bites, ringworm, athlete's foot, candida and genitourinary tract infections, gum and mouth infections, nausea, vomiting, diarrhoea, dysentery and as an antiseptic wash for cuts and grazes.

Bergamot is a sweet orange smelling oil. Apart from neroli, which is very expensive, it is the first choice for stress and anxiety. It is soothing for the nervous system and uplifting for the mind. It can both stimulate and sedate. It is one of the most valuable oils for improving one's psychological state. It is also helpful in urinary tract infections. (Avoid using any citrus oils if you are in the sun as they can cause uneven skin patches). Geranium is the most balancing of oils and helpful for women to balance their moods especially when the hormones are fluctuating around the time of menstruation or during menopause. It has a tonic effect on the liver and kidneys. Lavender, bergamot and geranium combined together make a balancing anti-stress oil.

Rosemary has a stimulating effect on the brain and nervous system but should be used sparingly and not used by people who have epilepsy. It is a good pick me up oil and clears the head when you feel tired or unclear after a late night or need to improve your concentration. It is good for relieving muscular pain or overworked muscles. Although it is considered to be a morning oil due to its stimulating effects, it can also be used in the bath at night to relax the muscles after a tiring day. Thyme is a natural antibiotic and has antiviral and diuretic properties. It should be used sparingly as it is very strong and can over stimulate. Eucalyptus has many medical properties including being antiviral. It can safely be used in a steam vaporizer or electric oil burner as a decongestant in a child or adult's room as an effective remedy for coughs and colds. (Never leave unattended oil burners with candles in a child's room.). It also prevents the spread of infection.

Four special oils for women are neroli, rose, jasmine and damiana. These four essential oils are considered to be spiritual oils that work both on the emotional and subtler levels of the body. They can be used individually or combined together as an exotic, uplifting and inspiring blend for women. However these oils are very expensive and for that reason they are usually only purchased by aromatherapists. Neroli is the first choice for stress and emotional imbalances. Rose is a woman's oil; it brings healing to the heart chakra. It is also suitable also for all disorders and imbalances of the reproductive system.

Jasmine is an exotic oil and wonderful when combined with damiana, they are both aphrodisiacs. Damiana is one of my favourite oils and combines beautifully with many other oils, it is a well sought after oil and not easy to find. It is helpful for premenstrual tension and stress and can be used as a tonic during and after menopause. It stimulates the pituitary gland and has an uplifting effect on the libido. Jasmine is also valuable as a uterine tonic for menstrual pain, during labour for relieving pain and cramps and a natural way to increase contractions. It is a helpful oil to use after childbirth if there is depression or postnatal blues. Rose is too expensive to be used in a burner but rosewood can be used instead. Rosewood is a lovely sweet, feminine oil, which encourages positive thought forms and combines well with Frankincense for meditation. It is said to be a healer of scar tissue, both physical and emotional.

Juniper is the oil to use both for physical and emotional detoxification. Add one or two drops (diluted in a teaspoon of almond oil) to the bath water either alone or with other oils and soak and release. Juniper and geranium have a cleansing and balancing effect and are a good combination during menstruation. Juniper is also recommended for cleansing the energies of the house or for clearing negative energies. Sage and cedarwood can also be used for cleaning the house.

Mandarin is good when doing inner child work. Elemi is a powerful oil for releasing blocked emotions, it can be used to activate the healing process and can bring clarity whilst doing inner work and visualizations. It combines well with lavender and a drop of juniper. Palmarosa is another sweet feminine oil, which is balancing and healing and helps where communication is blocked.

Frankincense, myrrh and benzoin are considered to be sacred oils. Frankincense has been used in temples and in the Catholic Church throughout the ages. It purifies the space and has a spiritually elevating influence. It brings the mind and body into a meditative state and is also considered to be a rejuvenating oil. Myrrh is used in Tibetan medicine for relieving stress and nervous disorders. As a spiritual oil, it is said to open the spiritual doorway, add just 1 drop to a blend or burner. Benzoin is an oil that gets things moving, it helps move both physical and energy blocks. It is a comforting oil and smells wonderful in the burner especially when mixed with Frankincense and bergamot. Benzoin is used in the Greek Orthodox church to purify and lift the vibrations. These three oils combined together create a wonderful synergy suitable for meditation and deep healing work.

Essential oils, which help with detoxification, are juniper, which is a diuretic and eliminates toxins from the urinary tract, kidneys and bladder. When combined with lemon, it helps release lymphatic congestion. Lemon also counteracts acidity. Sandalwood helps with urinary tract infections and thyme is useful for yeast and fungal infections including candida.

The following citrus oils are uplifting as well as inexpensive and therefore ideal to use in an oil burner. Choose from orange, lemon, lemongrass, mandarin, lime and grapefruit. Grapefruit helps clear negative energy (combine with juniper) and uplifts one's mood and detoxifies and cleanses the body and boosts a sluggish lymph system. (Add a few drops to the bath especially when feeling exhausted)

It is wonderful to burn essential oils whilst you sleep. Choose from lavender, bergamot, orange, rosewood or chamomile. Clary sage induces vivid dreams and helps us to remember our dreams. You can combine one or two drops with other oils. Never use Clary sage if you have drunk any alcohol as it can have the opposite effect and create nightmares. If you have any breathing problems or feel a cold coming on use eucalyptus oil, you only need a couple of drops because it is very strong.

Clary sage, lavender and juniper have a cleansing effect and can be used together for an evening, healing bath. Clary sage is also a phyto-oestrogen and is therefore good for use during menopause. Ginger increases the digestive fire and can be added to a bath for people who have bad circulation including cold hands and feet. It is recommended for morning sickness, nausea and slow digestion.

Flower Essences

Flower remedies or essences as they are most often called, work in a gentle and subtle, yet profound way. They are made from a highly diluted, water based extract of the vibration of the flower or plant. They are completely pure and there is no way you can overdose on them. If you select an incorrect remedy, it just won't work for you. Flower essences are an aspect of vibrational medicine; they resonate and rebalance the emotional, psychological, subtle energy system and spiritual aspects of our being. This does not mean we can just sit back and take flower essences, this is not the case, we still have to do the work of emotional clearing, but flower essences can greatly aid the process.

There are thousands of flower essences available, which can make it difficult to choose, which ones to use. You will have to experiment and see which ones work best for you, trust your intuition if you are drawn to a particular range of essences or an individual one. Kinesiology or dowsing with a pendulum are the best ways to select for yourself. I test myself every day with Kinesiology and select accordingly. I especially like the Himalayan flower essences and the Australian Bush essences. Both of these are very potent and come from areas where they is a lot of prana, high energy and exposure to the sun, which are essential ingredients for potent essences.

Dr. Bach's flower remedies are probably the most well known especially Rescue Remedy which is very helpful in any emergency especially for shock, stress and fear, also after operations. It can safely be given to babies, children and animals. Australian Bush essences also make an Emergency Essence and Findhorn have a First Aid Essence.

I like to work with the Himalayan Flower Enhancers, I find they are beautiful essences for women and promote wholeness and balance. There are few places on the earth where the life force is as strong, pure and vibrant as the Himalayas and where the earth pulsates with so much life force energy. These are called enhancers rather than remedies or essences because they help bring out what is already there. They help bring forth the true nature of the person and release what is blocking the true self from emerging. They have a useful set of eight chakra enhancers, which help activate and clear each of the chakras. I recommend people use one chakra essence for a period of a week beginning first with the base chakra and working upwards and then repeating the process. This helps bring balance throughout the whole system. Individual chakra enhancers can be used when needed.

Other Himalayan Flower Enhancers are Lotus, which is a symbol of enlightenment. It enhances the crown chakra and is useful in meditation and all forms of healing. It boosts all other herbs, and essences and is a general tonic and cleanser for the entire system. White Orchid open the higher aspect of the heart after emotional clearing work has been done and it enhances love and acceptance. Isan is from the flowers of the Neem tree and helps integrate mind, body and spirit. Goddess enhances the goddess energy and helps the feminine aspect and the wise woman to come forth.

Gulaga is powerful for clearing away issues from the past that are no longer relevant. Nirjana is useful for deconditioning on a cellular level, to release negative vibrations and reprogramme. Nirjana 2 helps decondition on a mental level, releasing mental thought forms and attitudes, which are not uplifting. Gateway assists in periods of transition or uncertainty and inner turmoil. Golden dawn aids women to release feelings of holding and being wounded in relation to sexuality. Children's Flower is an enhancer especially for children, to enhance their joy and playfulness, to protect them and to help them release anything that is disturbing them. Morning Glory reduces nervous tension and helps break addictions such as coffee, cigarettes and sugar.

The Australian Bush Essences make several good combination essences. Cognis Essence promotes mental clarity and focus. Dynamis encourages vitality, enthusiasm and a zest for life. Purifying Essence helps clear emotional overload.

Women's Essence aids women who are going though life changes and cycles including menopause. Emergency Essence is for emotional difficulties and has also been recommended for hot flushes. Travel Essence is a useful remedy for travellers and helps with jet lag and disorientation after travelling.

Findhorn Life Force combination essence helps revitalise and strengthen emotionally.

Perelandra rose essences are useful for grounding and integrating after spiritual experiences.

6 - MENSTRUATION, MENOPAUSE AND HORMONES

Over the last fifteen to twenty years there has been a huge increase in hormone related problems. Many women experience menstrual and reproductive problems including premenstrual tension, cramps, pain, heavy blood flow, irritability, moodiness, depression, infertility, fibroids and cysts. Also ovarian, uterine and breast cancer are on the increase. Very few male doctors or gynaecologists really understand or are truly sympathetic to the fluctuations and problems caused by imbalances in the female endocrine system. They often take a quick fix approach, which is to either give a pill or cut something out.

Women have to learn to monitor and understand their own cycles in order to be more in touch with their bodies and to be able to balance their hormones and to prepare themselves for menopause. I would advise any young women who are reading this not to skip over the information on menopause because the more aware you are of your menstrual cycles and what affects them, the more prepared you will be and the easier it will be to balance your hormones when you go through premenopause and menopause.

Good hormone production and hormone flow are essential for good health. Insufficient flow or the overproduction of hormones by any of the glands will imbalance that particular area and affect the other glands too. There is an important link between the hormones and the nervous system. The hormones are affected by the fluctuations of your emotions, stress and too fast, chaotic lifestyles. One of the reasons for the increase in hormonal imbalances nowadays is due to the large amount of hormones that are found in meat and dairy products. There is also thought to be a connection between the hormones in meat and dairy products and breast and uterine cancer.

Some gynaecologists who are aware of the dangers, advise their patients who are trying to get pregnant or who are pregnant to refrain from eating any red meat and to keep dairy products to a minimum to avoid the consumption of excess hormones and antibiotics and other medicines which are given to animals and that could be dangerous to the foetus. This may be one of the major factors contributing to the increase in menstrual problems and infertility. There are many herbs, which can be very helpful for the menstrual cycle and menopause.

Some women are lucky enough to move through the monthly cycle without hardly noticing it, whereas for others it can be a frustrating and difficult time of the month which leaves them feeling tired and emotionally drained. By getting to know your monthly cycles, you can plan around them. In some cultures such as in the Ayurvedic tradition and American Indian tribes, the woman is allowed to rest and rebalance during her menstrual cycle. She would not do any cooking or housework, the other women in the family would take over for her.

Today, this is not only impossible for most busy working women but would probably even be thought of as making an unnecessary fuss. This is because the process of menstruation is not honoured or respected, as it should be. During menstruation, the body wants to slow down and rest more, whilst purification takes place. During the first one or two days of menstruation and especially if there is a heavy blood flow, try to do as little as possible, let things wait, avoid doing lots of housework or heavy manual work or strenuous exercise. Try to rest more, have early nights and avoid stress. This will make a lot of difference to your cycle in the long run. Also avoid drinking alcohol and coffee during those days as they are dehydrating and make symptoms worse.

If you suffer from premenstrual tension, check out how many days before your cycle this usually occurs and treat yourself at this time to a healing session, reflexology or massage, it can make all the difference; plan it as your monthly treat. Rescue Remedy flower essence by Dr. Bach can be useful if you are feeling irritable and also rose oil is very soothing. Monitor your emotional ups and downs, so that you can see what is due to your monthly cycle or what is stress caused by other things. When you get clear, you can plan well around it, and take the necessary measures to move through this time more harmoniously and relaxed. If you feel moody due to hormone changes, explain it to your partner or boyfriend, so that they do not take it personally, it is hard for men to understand how a woman's hormones affect her moods but if they know it is not their fault, it makes things easier. The moon can also affect your monthly cycle, as can seasonal changes. Some women feel more irritable if their period coincides with the full moon cycle, whereas others can feel totally depleted if their period occurs around new moon.

If your monthly cycle is irregular, or you suffer from ups and downs or moodiness, one of the best herbs to take is Brazilian ginseng also known as pfaffia. It is a tonic for the reproductive cycle and helps stabilize the cycle or balance when periods are irregular. It is also helpful if the blood flow is scanty or too heavy. The other herb, which is very good for the reproductive system is Agnus Castus, which helps uterine pain or cramps during menstruation. Both of these herbs should be taken for a period of at least six months to see an ongoing improvement. It takes time to rebalance the hormones.

If you have a heavy blood flow, you have to watch your iron levels so as not to become depleted or anaemic. Premenstrual tension is sometimes associated with low iron levels. Rather than taking iron supplements, which often upset the stomach and are difficult for the body to assimilate, it is better to eat iron rich foods such as black molasses, raisins, oatmeal, green vegetables, seaweeds, whole wheat bread and grapes and to drink carrot juice, lapacho and dandelion tea.

Some women get strong headaches or even migraines before menstruation. If the headache is hormone related or because of blocked energy, guarana can quickly relieve the headache. Rubbing the back of the neck and forehead with lavender oil can also help alleviate a headache. When the menstrual flow is heavy avoid hot baths, massage and strenuous exercise, let the body rest and cleanse.

Many women have sweet cravings just before or during the days of their menstruation, try to avoid white flour and white sugar products which make the symptoms worse and instead choose natural sweeteners like honey, dried fruits and fresh fruit juices to satisfy the sweet craving.

Menopause

Menopause is a natural process that women go through when their menstrual cycle stops and brings about a change in metabolism. In most women this change occurs somewhere between their late forties to early fifties. Menopause is not an illness, it is a natural body process and except for rare cases there should be no need for replacement therapy or the taking of hormones, which interfere with the natural flow of hormone production. It is unnatural to prolong the menstrual cycle through taking chemicals; this creates an imbalance in the endocrine system. The body knows when it is time to stop; menopause is a natural phase of a woman's reproductive cycle, the same as puberty and the onset of menstruation and the less interference the better.

The first signs of menopause begin with a change in the menstrual cycle, usually the periods start to become irregular and there may be months when they are missed altogether and this may then be followed by a period of heavy bleeding and the release of blood clots. This is usually nothing to worry about and a normal part of the change. The irregularity of the menstrual cycle may continue for a few months or years. The average age to stop is 51. It is important to wait until 13-14 months after the last period before discontinuing the use of contraception. Some women have been known to get pregnant a few months after there last period. After menstruation stops completely, the hormones will still keep adjusting for the next five to ten years so it is important to maintain one's balance and rest sufficiently and avoid stress and strain during this time so as to pave the way for maintaining good health in the latter years of life.

Depending on how you have taken care of yourself and your health, will determine how your body will respond during menopause. The more settled and balanced you are during the years of premenopause, the easier the transition of menopause will be. Some women sail through menopause without any discomfort, hardly noticing anything and wondering what all the fuss is about; others have a hard time and experience many symptoms of discomfort. Most women fall into the category that is somewhere in between. Women who are smokers or who have been heavy smokers may have an earlier menopause or more difficult menopausal symptoms.

The most common symptoms of menopause are irregular periods, heavy blood flow, hot flushes, night sweats, vaginal dryness, irritability, low libido, lack of sex drive, dry skin, weight gain, headaches, mood swings, depression and low energy. The two most common symptoms which many women experience are hot flushes and night sweats. Although these can be uncomfortable, they are both harmless. Hot flushes and night sweats increase if you are run down, exhausted or stressed. Irregular sleep patterns, sleeping late, eating heavy late meals or drinking alcohol including wine make hot flushes and night sweats worse. If you do experience either of these symptoms, then it is best to avoid all heating foods including garlic, onion, ginger, hot peppers, spicy and sour foods including vinegar. Don't eat very hot food or drink hot beverages, allow them to cool. Also avoid hot baths, saunas or sitting in the sun, as these increase the heat in the body.

The most useful and popular herb, which I have found for women going through menopause and can be taken during and after menopause is pfaffia. It is a natural hormone balancer, tonic and food supplement for the reproductive system. It is an adaptogen, which means that it helps the body either increase or decrease hormone levels according to the needs of the body through naturally balancing the hormones. It is considered one of the most effective alternatives to HRT and helpful with the symptoms of menopause.

If the hot flushes are still very strong after a month or two on pfaffia, you can combine it with black cohash tincture for a couple of months and then go back to taking only pfaffia. Sage also helps reduce hot flushes and night sweats but should not be taken for long periods of time. Mint tea, fennel tea or water with a squeeze of fresh lemon juice (no sugar) have cooling properties. Cumin is a cooling spice, which can be added to cooking. Aloe vera juice is a blood purifier and has a cooling and pacifying effect. Raisins are healthy and cooling, take 2-3 tablespoons with your food every day. Regular kidney cleansing with quebra pedra tea, liver detoxification, coffee enemas and colonics are cleansing and heat reducing.

On a metaphysical level hot flushes are associated with heat rising in the body from the energy vortex at the base of the spine, known as the kundalini. This sometimes gets activated in women around menopause and may be experienced as waves of heat rising up through the body. This is an awakening process that should not be suppressed. When a woman allows herself to move through this experience naturally, then after the completion of menopause, her intuition or sixth sense can be activated and the wise woman in her can be awakened.

In certain traditions, this time is considered very sacred for a woman and it is only after having completed menopause that a woman may be allowed to engage in higher spiritual practises. Taking hormone replacement therapy interferes with this natural process and confuses both the normal production of hormones and the energy system and prevents the deeper aspects of the woman from awakening and this can cause deep emotional frustration. Menopause is a time for a woman to honour herself and welcome a new phase of maturity that will bring deeper wisdom, new insights and a new phase of life.

Sometimes during menopause there may be sporadic heavy bleeding caused by fibroids, which are non-malignant growths in the uterus. Most fibroids and cysts disappear without intervention after menopause. There is a tendency to recommend hysterectomy for almost any gynaecological problem around menopause, doctors often advise removal of the ovaries, just to be on the safe side; in most cases this is not necessary. Recent research has shown that as high as three out of four hysterectomies were not really necessary. Before making a final decision, get a second or even third opinion and investigate other options such as seeing a natural practitioner, Ayurvedic doctor or medical herbalist before making a decision. Unless the situation is life threatening, don't make quick decisions to get it over and done with, there may be complications afterwards and the recovery time might be from three to six months or even longer as the body tries to adjust. A hysterectomy is major surgery, all surgery is invasive and should be seen as a last resort. Keeping your ovaries is important for your long-term health as the ovaries continue to secrete hormones even after menopause.

There are many things a woman can do for herself to balance her hormones and to make the transition smoother. Many women feel depressed because they see it as the end of their life because they are getting old. This does not happen for instance in indigenous tribes where the elders are highly respected for their wisdom, which has been gained through life experiences. Menopause is an opportunity to embrace the changes that are happening, to acknowledge that you are moving into a new phase of your life and to welcome it. This is a time to start something new, to find new channels of interest and especially the time to begin exploring the spiritual path and allowing the spiritual woman to emerge.

During menopause, you need to take extra care to nourish yourself on every level, to eat and sleep well and to keep stress to a minimum in order to assist your body in the best possible way through this time of transition. The more you nourish yourself, the better you will feel. Try to avoid stress and anything that may imbalance you emotionally, this is a time for stability, balance and harmony. It is a time to honour and pamper yourself.

Reflexology is a very supportive treatment during menopause. If you have regular treatments during this time, it will help balance the whole body including the hormones and special attention can be given to the ovaries and uterus. It also helps with cleansing and detoxification and improves circulation and the function of all the organs. Reflexology is very relaxing and if you find a therapist who combines reflexology with healing, this takes the process deeper. Being a reflexologist myself, I know the value of the treatments. I had reflexology sessions every week for a year whilst going through menopause and I felt that it helped keep me balanced; it was a gift to myself. Gentle massage such as aromatherapy can also be enjoyable but avoid deep massage during this time and instead choose treatments that are gentle, healing and nurturing. There are special oils, which can be used during this time, my favourite is a Maharishi Ayurvedic combination of oils called Transition.

Sometimes women get worried because they seem to lose interest in sex during menopause, they may not have the energy for it because the body needs a lot of energy to adjust to the hormonal changes that are taking place. This is usually only temporary and herbs such as damiana help improve libido and pfaffia helps with the problem of dry vagina, which can make sexual intercourse painful.

During menopause it is recommend to include soya products in the diet such as tofu and soya milk, which contain a hormonal type substance called genostein, which can help reduce hot flushes. In Japan where they eat a lot of soya products, women rarely experience hot flushes. Soya milk is high in protein and equivalent to the amount of calcium found in milk or other dairy products. It contains estrogenic properties, which are helpful for menopausal women but it should be drunk only in small amounts and not be drunk by breast-feeding mothers or by women who have a problem with too much oestrogen in their bodies and it should not given to children There has been some question recently about soya products due to the fact that some soya beans are genetically engineered, so choose either organic soya milk or companies that state that there products are not genetically engineered.

Avoid estrogenic chemicals which imbalance the endocrine system, these include canned foods, preservatives, synthetic hormones, pesticides and fertilizers. They stimulate the over production of hormones, which is one of the causes of cysts, cancer, tumours and weight gain. Instead increase your intake of fresh plant foods, which are rich in phytoestrogens and help balance the endocrine system. Doctors don't know about the wonderful power of plants during menopause, that is why many of them automatically prescribe HRT without investigating other more natural possibilities.

Include daily helpings of salads, fresh vegetables, fruits and lentils. Phytoestrogens are foods that contain plant hormones which naturally balance the hormonal system, these include mung beans, chick peas, (include lots of pulses) peas, broccoli, celery, brazil nuts, tahini, linseeds, sesame, pumpkin and sunflower seeds, alfalfa and mung bean sprouts, almonds, dried figs, parsley and fennel. Including lots of phytoestrogens in your diet lowers the risk of breast cancer. Also include many of the foods from the Superfoods list. Liquorice root powder is an adaptogen which helps decrease or increase oestrogen levels according to the body's needs. Other foods to eat are dates, oats, bananas, green beans, rye, yam, honey, avocado, apples, grapes and citrus fruits. It is recommended to eat oatmeal (porridge) once a day; it is high in vitamin B, good for the bones and very nourishing and balancing for menopausal women. Add dried fruits, honey, ghee and chopped almonds to oatmeal with soya milk to increase stamina. Add lots of ghee to your food as it is balancing and purifying.

Linseeds are an essential food to help prevent dry, flaking skin, dandruff and dry vagina, which are often associated with menopause. Linseeds, also known as flaxseeds contain an oestrogenically active compound which helps produce strong bones, nails and teeth and protect against breast cancer. These little seeds are highly beneficial during menopause and have been classed as a miracle food because they contain all the necessary essential fatty acids and are also antiviral, antifungal, antibacterial and also good for constipation. Add one or two tablespoons every day to your breakfast cereal or sprinkle on salads or vegetables. Essential fatty acids lubricate the joints, skin and vagina and help prevent blood clots and keep the blood thin. A deficiency in EFA results in dry skin, lifeless hair, cracked nails, fatigue, aching joints and arthritis. You can also take starflower oil or evening primrose supplements, which are high in EFA. Other sources of EFA are nuts and seeds especially almonds, brazil nuts and walnuts. Daily sesame oil massage is recommended to feed and lubricate the skin and joints.

Herb teas to drink during this time are damiana, a wonderful woman's tea, which stimulates the libido and fennel, which has a similar effect. Chamomile, orange blossom and lime blossom, balm and passionflower are all relaxing and soothing teas and good to drink in the evening. Dandelion is good for general detoxification and lapacho tea stimulates the immune system. A high-powered energy breakfast food can be made from a combination of dried dates, figs, raisins and prunes, which have been soaked overnight and then blended with the water they were soaked in, then add crushed almonds, honey, ghee, a pinch of liquorice and vanilla. This is delicious, nourishing and energizing.

Two other herbs, which are useful during menopause and discussed more in detail in the chapter on Nature's Gifts are guarana, which can be taken when there is a lack of energy, moodiness or depression and ginkgo biloba for fogginess in the mind, lack of concentration or memory. Noni is a juice from Tahiti, which helps the heart through purifying the blood and maintaining regular blood pressure and cleansing the cells. It is considered to be anti cancerous. It has an overall balancing effect; it rebalances blood pressure, sugar levels and the hormones. It is good to take every day as a general tonic.

The right type of gentle exercise is very important during menopause, nothing too strenuous but enough to keep the energy flowing and to increase circulation of the blood and lymph so as to assist the body whilst it rebalances and adjusts to the hormonal changes. Yoga is very beneficial during menopause, it helps the body to readjust and to rebalance the hormones and it also calms the nervous system and relieves stress. It has been described as a gift for all ages but especially as a gift for old age because you can continue practising Yoga until any age. Yoga promotes better blood circulation and oxygenation of the cells and increases metabolism and energy flow. Yoga also maintains flexibility of the spine, which supports all systems and increases youthfulness and prevents premature ageing.

Pranayama breathing exercises and relaxation, which are included in Yoga sessions, help ease mood swings and depression and alleviate anxiety, which may be experienced during the change. Pelvic floor exercises strengthen the pelvic area and increase circulation and blood supply to the pelvic area and can help tighten the vagina and prevent dryness. Building up the muscles through lightweight training is also important.

After menopause we start to age faster as the metabolism slows down, so we need all the help we can get and everything that has been mentioned regarding diet and lifestyle is very important at this time. Regular exercise, eating less and detoxification, all help improve metabolism. Lots of walking is good for the circulation and the heart. It is natural to gain some weight during menopause so don't be obsessed with being thin, accept the natural changes of your body and love and nurture yourself.

Menopause can be an emotional time; emotions can be very strong especially if you have been suppressing them or not expressing yourself enough. If you are experiencing lots of emotional ups and downs, get support. Talking, sharing and deep emotional release work is very important during this transitional time. Rebirthing combined with healing, which will be discussed in greater detail is a wonderful way of doing this and can clear layers of resentment and frustration from the past and allow a new self to emerge. Heated emotions such as anger and rage can increase hot flushes and night sweats. Suppressing them will only make you feel worse, releasing them in a safe, comfortable situation such as during rebirthing, can be freeing and give a deep sense of relief. Do not expect your doctor if he is male or your partner to really understand what you are going through, most likely they won't, getting the support of other women who have been through the change can be very supportive.

Hormone Replacement Therapy

When hormone replacement therapy first appeared on the market, it was hailed as a wonder drug for women and seen as the answer to many menopausal symptoms and even an antidote to ageing. As with all new experimental drugs, it takes ten to fifteen years before the side effects of a drug become evident and unfortunately it has now been seen that HRT has many unpleasant side effects including increased risk of endometrial and breast cancer, vaginal bleeding, blood clots and cysts and 70% increased risk of heart attack, weight gain, sore breasts, fluid retention, depression, insomnia, liver dysfunction, headaches and increase of body hair. Over half the women who take HRT stop after three months because of the uncomfortable side effects. Although some women find that their symptoms are greatly relieved whilst on HRT, as soon as they stop taking it the symptoms come back often even stronger, which shows that it does nothing to help with the underlying imbalances, it only temporarily suppresses them.

Taking chemical hormones confuses the body's natural intelligence by interfering with natural hormone production. There are many ways of bringing the body back to balance in a natural way, without putting yourself at risk to the dangerous side effects of HRT. This is a choice that every woman has to make for herself. Because of the dangers, women on HRT need to be screened more often for breast and uterine cancer.

One of the arguments for HRT and the reason why many women take it is because it was believed that it might be helpful in protecting the bones and preventing osteoporosis. There are however no proven studies or scientific evidence to back this. Recent results of studies in Massachusetts's show that HRT fails to protect women from osteoporosis and that women on HRT also get osteoporosis. Some reports claimed that bone mass could be preserved after HRT had been taken for ten to fifteen years but as soon as it was stopped the mineral density declines rapidly. Most women in their fifties and sixties are not at risk but women in their seventies and eighties are and may suffer hip or other bone fractures This means that they would have to take HRT for thirty years but it is not advised to stay on HRT more than one or two years. The longer HRT is used, the greater the risk of breast and endometrical cancer.

Do not feel pressurized into taking HRT because of fear of osteoporosis. Instead pay more attention to your diet and lifestyle, listen to your body and make the necessary changes. There are home urine evaluation tests, which you can do which are safer than bone scans and exposure to harmful x-rays. Some bio resonance programmes can also effectively and safely scan the bones. The most effective prevention is a change in diet and lifestyle and choosing natural supplements rather than taking a drug that is made from pregnant horses' urine.

Nowadays many doctors are more aware of the dangers and are more cautious about giving HRT to their patients and encourage them instead to choose more natural ways of maintaining their hormone levels. In some countries, by law doctors have to fully inform their patients of all the possible risks in taking HRT before prescribing it. This year, in August 2002, the National Cancer Institute reported that post-menopausal women who take oestrogen for ten years or more have a full 60% higher risk of developing ovarian cancer than women who never take it. The negative impact of these studies has shocked many doctors and women, who are now seriously considering what other measures can be taken.

If you are considering taking HRT, discuss the possible side effects and dangers with your doctor, read more on the subject and then decide if it is worth it. Evaluate how serious your symptoms are and look into alternative methods of balancing your hormones rather than taking a quick fix when you experience discomfort. HRT is often given to women with only mild symptoms or just in case, the risks are far too great and if you do have to take it for serious complications then try not to stay on it more than a year or two. Remember that menopause is a natural process, the body knows how to rebalance itself but this takes time and it is not natural to prolong menstruation, the body knows when it is time to stop.

Although many doctors are investigating alternatives and working alongside with natural practitioners, there are just as many who are too busy and do not have the time to read up on the latest information that is available. What they don't know, they cannot recommend. Women doctors tend to be more open in incorporating alternatives and complimentary treatments. Explore your choices carefully, read as much as possible, talk to other women and go to women's wellness centres and natural health centres to learn more about what is available and get emotional support when you need it.

Osteoporosis

Osteoporosis is a disorder of progressive bone loss; the bones become brittle, thin and porous and break easily. Bone loss results when the rate of renewal does not equal the rate of breakdown. In the last ten to fifteen years there has been a dramatic increase in osteoporosis, it is estimated that one in four women in the western world over the age of fifty may develop osteoporosis. This is very high and a cause for great concern. The good news is that osteoporosis can be prevented and bones can be rebuilt through correct nutrition and exercise.

The main causes of osteoporosis are a lack of calcium and a lack of oestrogen and eating large amounts of milk and dairy products. In African countries where they don't eat dairy products or a lot of refined sugar, they do not have osteoporosis. Consuming too much sugar, caffeine, alcohol and smoking leeches calcium from the bones. Calcium depletion and bone loss begin in mid life and are not due to menopause but to a combination of factors including poor diet, stress, over exercising or not exercising enough and leading a sedentary lifestyle, strain, anorexia and high toxicity and acidity levels. Thinning bones have less to do with menopause than with Western dietary practices and can largely be prevented by diet and regular exercise. Taking tranquilizers, sleeping pills and too many pharmaceutical medicines increase the risk factors.

The amount of oestrogen in the body fluctuates during menopause but this is natural and not the major cause of the problem, although women who have an early menopause are seen to be more at risk for osteoporosis because of lower oestrogen levels in the body for many years. Pfaffia, Brazilian ginseng has already been mentioned as one of the best herbs to help maintain natural hormone levels and balance and helps the body to produce more oestrogen when needed. Gradual bone loss can begin ten to fifteen years before menopause. Bones have the ability to renew themselves; so the earlier you start a prevention programme the better, prevention is always better than cure. You can greatly reduce the risk of osteoporosis by not smoking and avoiding alcohol, sugar, coffee, cola drinks and red meat. Refined white sugar interferes with the absorption of calcium and magnesium. Caffeine and dairy products draw calcium out of the bones.

Strong bones need a diet that includes an adequate amount of calcium and is rich in minerals including magnesium, potassium and zinc. They also benefit from good circulation, assimilation and a strong metabolism, regular exercise and keeping toxicity and acidity levels to a minimum. Genetic and hereditary factors are most often attributed to having the same lifestyle habits and preferences as parents and other family members. Daily exercise is recommended to maintain bone mass such as walking, swimming, dancing, Yoga and gentle weight bearing exercise. Over exercising or strenuous exercise is not recommended after the late 40s because it can increase bone loss. Yoga helps build up bone density and strength and it is recommended to do at least fifteen to twenty minutes Yoga every day.

About ten years ago, there was a protein myth circulating and doctors thought that eating lots of animal protein might be helpful for the bones, now the opposite has been proved that people who eat too much animal protein are more susceptible to softening and weakening of the bones, which leads to the bones becoming more fragile and fractures and osteoporosis. Research shows that vegetarians who eat a healthy, mineral rich diet with lots of fruits and vegetables and eat only very little animal protein tend to have stronger bones and higher bone density and therefore less bone fractures and less osteoporosis. It is important to nourish and feed the bones well. Avoid taking foods which are acidic and rob the body of calcium by keeping red meat and hard cheeses to a minimum or better still cut them out altogether and drastically reduce the intake of sugar, white flour products, refined foods, alcohol including wine, coffee, tea and fizzy drinks which all draw calcium from the bones and interfere with calcium absorption. Avoid salt and add herbs and spices to food instead.

Foods, which have the highest calcium content and should be regularly included in your diet, are tofu, soya milk, tahini, sesame seeds and almonds. Other calcium rich foods are sunflower seeds, dried figs, brazil nuts, broccoli, mung beans, chickpeas and dark green leafy vegetables (careful of eating too much spinach which is acidic). Dandelion is high in calcium, so drink one cup of dandelion tea a day. Rose lassi is very nourishing and a good daily source of calcium and can be eaten with food. Put one third to half a cup of fresh, live yogurt with the same amount of water, 2 teaspoons rosewater, 1 teaspoon of honey and 1 teaspoon of linseed oil or mint if preferred rather than the sweet taste and mix well together. Avoid yoghurts which are mixed with fruit, these cause fermentation because fruit and dairy don't mix well. Vitamin D is necessary for calcium absorption and healthy bones. Your skin manufactures vitamin D when it is exposed to sunlight, vitamin D is also found in fish oils and cereals.

During menopause, it is important to increase your supply of minerals by eating oatmeal, seaweeds or kelp (for iodine), black molasses, lots of green leafy vegetables especially broccoli. Take one to two tablespoons of aloe vera juice daily, which is full of minerals. Apple cider vinegar is also rich in minerals and has a cleansing effect. Take 1 to 2 teaspoons of cider vinegar with 1 teaspoon of honey in warm water first thing in the morning as a general tonic. Fennel tea is very rich in minerals and is known to be helpful for osteoporosis as it feeds the bones as well as maintaining the elasticity of the skin and connective tissue. Dried apricots contain boron, which is needed for strong bones; soak them overnight to make their easily digestible. We need calcium for the hard tissue and potassium for the soft tissue, magnesium is another mineral, which is essential for the bones and is necessary for the absorption of calcium. For foods, which are rich in calcium, boron, magnesium and iron see the Conscious Eating chapter. It is also good to include lots of grains in your diet to protect your bones, include basmati rice, semolina, couscous and oats.

There is an important connection between acidity and dry, brittle bones. When there is an acidic environment within the body, calcium is pulled out of the bones. It is important for the maintenance of healthy bones to create a more alkaline environment within the body. For proper functioning of our metabolism, the blood needs to be slightly alkaline. Lots of minerals in the blood alkalise the body. A build up of uric acid causes arthritis as well as osteoporosis. Many degenerative diseases including cancer are linked to over acidity. A healthy body has calcium reserves in the body but over acidity draws calcium from the bones to compensate. The level of PH, the acid or alkaline level in the body, can be determined by a simple litmus paper test at home. 7.2 is normal, lower means there is acidity. I always test my clients for acidity because so often this lies at the root of many problems.

People who smoke or drink a lot of coffee, tea or alcohol usually have high acidity levels. Red meat is acidic and full of hormones. An alkaline diet, including lots of fruit, vegetables and grains, protects the bones and prevents calcium and minerals from being leeched from the bones. The combination of smoking, alcohol and coffee increase the possibility of brittle bones by 400%. Cleaning the kidneys regularly through drinking quebra pedra tea helps improve the functioning of the kidneys and urinary tract and the acid alkaline level of the body by removing acids from the urinary system. Too many acids in the body are the main cause of cystitis. Noni juice helps flush out the toxins and acids and is recommended on a daily basis as a tonic and for cellular detoxification. Inner and outer oleation of the body helps remove toxins and acids from the joints and bones. Give yourself a daily sesame oil massage and include olive oil, linseeds and ghee in your food on a daily basis and make sure to drink enough water, between eight to ten glasses a day to prevent dryness and brittleness of the bones. You can also take a combined supplement of evening primrose oil, borage oil and starflower oil, which is high in essential fatty acids.

It was discovered that the people living in Okinawa islands in Japan live long lives, some of the oldest people in the world live there and they are vibrant and healthy. The secret to their health lies in the water, which is infused with coral calcium that is very alkaline and has a PH value of 8.6. Alka-mine is pulverized coral calcium that is packaged in sachets like tea bags that can be added to water or other drinks. The high concentration of calcium and magnesium in the coral calcium feeds the bones in a natural way that can easily be absorbed by the body and corrects the acid alkaline balance by encouraging detoxification through the release of excess acids. It also contains many other minerals so it is a recommended supplement to take for healthy bones.

Cancer

Cancer is on the increase in women, especially breast and uterine cancer. Cancer can be life threatening and just the word brings up fear and dread. Many factors are involved in the development of cancer; there is most often a strong underlying emotional factor, either the suppression of feelings or an inability to cope with certain life situations or a lot of inner stress and tension. When this is combined with a weak immune system due to overuse of antibiotics and prescribed drugs, incorrect diet and high toxicity and acidity levels, then an unhealthy inner environment is created and the cells may begin to function abnormally and go out of control. This situation may be prevalent in the body for many years before it is pinpointed, that is why so often cervical smears and mammography scannings do not show up the cancerous cells. It is only when a large number of cancerous cells become evident, that they are identified in tests.

There is a known connection between cancer and smoking, cells that are starved of oxygen are more likely to become cancerous. Food also plays an important role in healthy cell development; the blood of cancer patients has been shown to be deficient in certain nutrients. Cancer cells thrive on sugar, which increases the production of lactic acid and creates an acidic environment that encourages the cancerous cells to reproduce faster and for the cancer cells to spread. Cancer is rare in countries where they eat natural foods and no processed foods or sugar, as soon as they adopt a western type diet and lifestyle including an increased consumption of sugar and a more stressful lifestyle, and then cancer starts to appear.

Cancer promoting foods include meat, which is high in hormones that are dangerous for human consumption and foods which may be cooked in rancid oils such as chips, crisps and roasted nuts, sugar, refined products, all unnatural products, processed, tinned, packed, frozen and precooked food, also microwave ovens have been linked with cancer. Low amounts of selenium in the soil and a lack of iodine have been associated with breast cancer. Being overweight is another risk factor for cancer.

Eating a cancer prevention diet with plenty of easily digestible foods is essential for everyone; include lots of fresh vegetable, fruits, pulses, salads and whole grains and plenty of the foods on the Superfoods list. Beta-carotene is an immune protector against cancer and is found in orange foods such as carrots, dried apricots and pumpkin.

Breast cancer is the most common form of cancer among women. Breast cancer has tripled in the last thirty years, and is the most prevalent five to ten years before menopause. Fifty per cent of women get breast lumps or breast cysts around premenopause due to too much oestrogen but most of these disappear after menopause. Most breast lumps are not malignant but it is always best to check them out to be on the safe side. High oestrogen levels and imbalanced hormone production are affected by stress, anger, negative emotions and a stressful lifestyle including not getting enough rest and early sleep. The risk factors increase for women who smoke, don't exercise regularly, and are overweight, stressed and eat lots of convenience foods including a high sugar or alcohol intake, which increases acidity. Other risk factors are if someone in the family had cancer, especially the mother, women who have never had children or had a late menopause, over the age of 55. Being very overweight after menopause also places a strain on the heart. Heart attacks amongst women are on the increase. Research is being made between the connection between dietary factors and drinking too much alcohol and breast cancer.

Wearing bras that are too tight or with wires underneath cuts off the lymph flow and can create blockages and cysts in the breasts. Try to go without wearing a bra as often as possible especially whenever you are at home. Most antiperspirants contain aluminium, which is poisonous and blocks the glands and can contribute to breast problems, instead choose natural deodorants that do not contain aluminium or crystal deodorant stones which are chemical free.

There is conflicting information on mammograms, breast cancer grows very slowly, by the time breast cancer is visible on a mammogram, it has been in the body for 6-7 years. Mammograms are commonly recommended but there are negative side effects from x-rays, which can contribute to breast cancer. Mammograms often give false readings, and women may be recalled, which means another dose of x-ray. Women who have regular mammograms every year fall into the high-risk group for breast cancer. From an esoteric perspective, breast cancer is most often associated with problems to do with relationships or heart issues such as feeling unloved or unappreciated or unfinished business such as resentment towards a partner or a relationship in the past that did not end well.

Deciding whether to have chemotherapy for cancer or to try alternatives is a very personal and often difficult decision. Chemotherapy greatly weakens the immune system and is very often unsuccessful; the cancer may come back and require second or third doses of chemotherapy making the immune system weaker and weaker or show up somewhere else. Deciding to go the alternative route takes courage and needs a lot of support. Two clinics that have done wonderful work with cancer using alternative methods and are worth investigating are the Gerson Institute in USA and the Bristol Cancer Clinic in UK. Whatever treatment you decide on, it can also be helpful to work with a healer at the same time. If you do decide on chemotherapy, healing treatments can minimalize the side effects of the treatments and support the immune system.

Lapacho (pau d arco) is a very good immune stimulant and lapacho tea is given with success to many cancer patients in Brazil. Research on Noni juice shows that it can normalize cancer cells. Essiac is a herbal mixture of American Indian origin, several books have been written on the benefits and healing effects of Essiac on cancer and other degenerative diseases. Graviola is a herb from the Amazon that is attracting a lot of attention. It is said to be effective in killing many different types of cancer cells, it hunts and destroys cancer cells without killing other cells. Research has recently been carried out by the National Cancer Institute on Graviola and it is likely that we will be hearing a lot more about this herb in the near future.

Maggie Erotokritou

PART 2

HEALING THE CAUSE

Maggie Erotokritou

7 - ESOTERIC HEALING

Throughout the ages there have been many esoteric schools, which were renowned for their teachings and exploration into the ancient wisdom of esoteric healing. Until recent years, these teachings were available only to the select few. In the past the knowledge was kept secret and only passed onto highly advanced practitioners in temples or healing circles. One could enter such circles only upon invitation and after passing through various initiations and tests. Today things are different; the ancient wisdom is being shared more openly and is available to anyone who is interested to learn.

Traditionally women were the healers, the carers, the nurturers and the wise women. Their intuition was more developed than men who lived primarily by their intellect. Every culture had its wise women and spiritual healers who knew the power of working with spirit and used the power of nature to heal. The Goddess culture revered and acknowledged the intuition, wisdom and healing power of women.

The fast changing role of the modern day woman living in a competitive world, has led to confusion about what a woman's role really is. As she tries to adapt and fulfil many aspects of herself as well as satisfying the demands that are made upon her by her family, work and the surrounding environment, she encounters many challenges. In the search and struggle for freedom and emancipation and the desire to become equal and accepted and to gain recognition, many women have lost their sense of the divine feminine and the feminine wisdom. They have unknowingly relinquished their inborn divine feminine power and wisdom and this has left them feeling unsatisfied and empty. There is a longing to heal the separation from the divine self. Reconnecting to the true self, the divinity within is the deepest healing that can take place, and through this we can find again the wholeness, happiness and peace that are a woman's natural birthright.

147

Women all over the world are reawakening to the wise woman within. That is why there has been such a recent surge of interest in spirituality, healing, natural medicine and anything connected to these fields. The power to heal is a woman's gift and can be given through a touch, a look or loving vibrations. Awakening to the feminine wisdom requires deep listening and observation, and the understanding that health and healing can only come when there is peace in the soul. As you learn more about your body and how it functions and watch your mind and observe your emotions and energy level, the wisdom will start to flow through.

There is nothing more powerful than the highly developed intuition of an awakened woman. Her intuition is sharp like a fine-tuning tool, she knows and she acts on her knowingness. Through awakening and developing the inner knowingness, you can spin a new web of life that is healthier, more vital and pregnant with possibilities. When your intuition is highly developed, you know the next step and each step leads to the next, you have a clearer sense of what you need to do and you draw the right people and circumstances to you.

The ancient teachings are based upon fundamental principles and natural laws, although specific methods and applications may vary. Each school has its particular system of healing, prayers, meditations and rituals but underneath there are similarities and connecting threads that link everything together. No matter which path you choose, all true seekers are moving in the same direction, towards self-realization and the expansion of consciousness, inner peace and happiness.

My own personal spiritual journey and exploration into healing started about twenty years ago. It began with Yoga and meditation and my training in Psychosynthesis, a transpersonal psychotherapy, where I trained as a therapist. This laid the foundation for the work, which was yet to come. I explored and became involved in many different systems and schools both in the fields of natural medicine and healing and the spiritual and esoteric. My travels to Tibet, India,

Nepal, Israel, Sinai and Morocco gave me deeper insights into the real value of life as well as enriching my knowledge about health, healing and consciousness. Each outer journey was in essence an inner journey that brought about profound shifts in consciousness and understanding.

Healing is an alchemical process of change and transformation, which takes place simultaneously on different levels. Through healing, imbalances and disharmony can be restored, stagnation can be removed, pain and obstructions can disappear and energy can be increased or decreased according to what is needed. The mind, body, emotions and spirit can be brought into alignment so as to function harmoniously together, so that radiant health and a higher level of existence can be experienced. People often think of healing in regards to just the physical body but in healing, the physical, mental, emotional and spiritual are seen as being intrinsically linked; what affects one will influence all the others. The aim is always to create balance, harmony and unity. The ageless wisdom taught that everything is interconnected and that nothing should be treated in isolation. Many of the alternative or complimentary therapies that are practised today, evolved from the roots of esoteric healing.

Healing is like a journey, moving from one state to another, from illness to health, from pain to joy, from inertia to wakefulness, from darkness into light and from ignorance to illumination. Healing is a learning process, which can affect and change every aspect of your life. It can be gentle and subtle, deep and profound or powerful and miraculous. Healing is not about a quick fix, although spontaneous and miraculous healings do occur, it is a process of change, learning and evolution.

In the ancient Yogic texts it is written that the root of illness begins in the mind and that the mind creates stresses, emotional disturbances and illusions. These misconceptions of the mind create imbalances, which lie at the root of ill health and unhappiness. Therefore we must also work with the mind in order to become aware of what we have created so as to heal and to see clearly the potential that lies behind everything. Any journey of exploration into healing begins in the present moment. By examining consciously what is present right now, what is your experience, how do you feel and what is the state of your health right now, will give you insights into what needs attention first, and what steps that you can take to make the necessary changes.

At your innermost core is the real self and as that part of you wakes up and becomes more aware, then every cell in your body wakes up too. Whatever you have programmed through your mind into the cells of your body has created your present state. Every thought, feeling and experience has an effect. All your life experiences and the affects of certain events in your life especially the difficult or more traumatic ones and the way you handled or rejected them are registered in your body. Your response, reaction or resistance to these experiences will indicate how much you were able to integrate, release and heal them or whether you are still holding and have suppressed or blocked your feelings.

If there are unresolved issues from the past or people you have not forgiven, this may interfere with the process of healing. Real healing comes from the core, from a place deep within that is truly accepting, forgiving, understanding and compassionate. We must look at the mental and emotional causes that lie behind imbalances and disease. If there is something that disturbs you, you need to go to the root of the problem and heal the wound. If you just leave it there and ignore it, then it may fester and create cancer or a tumour or some other physical problem. Deep emotional release work can be tranformative and enlightening, it can change us profoundly. As we let go and heal the past, we create the space and the opportunity for something new to come in. This frees up blocked energy, and can also release physical pain. (There will be more information on releasing emotional pain, traumas and past experiences in the chapters on The Wounded Woman and Rebirthing.)

Deep emotional release work is an important aspect of healing. Stress and emotional discord fragment us and make us imbalanced so that we lose our true sense of self. If we are not harmonious and balanced within, then how can we expect to interact in a harmonious way with others? A disturbed or irritated mind prevents us from seeing clearly and negative feelings will prevent healing from occurring. Your mental and emotional state bring about a corresponding state in your body and this affects the nervous system, the hormones, the immune system, the reproductive system, the organs and every other part of the body. By paying attention to your thoughts, emotions and energy level, as well as living a lifestyle that is supportive of creating radiant health, then healing and transformation can take place. Reprogramming and restructuring have to take place at the level of the DNA, which is also called the sacred memory. The body's inner intelligence has to be activated to assist the cellular reprogramming and to make the necessary changes.

Esoteric healing is about inner work; it moves us into the realms of self-development, self-actualisation and consciousness. It propels us to look deeper, to see what lies behind things, to find the real cause of imbalance and to address any emotional discord or discontent. Fear and resistance often come up when you are working on yourself and may prevent you from moving forward. At this point it can be helpful to get support or work with someone who will help you move through the blockages and assist you in letting go of the old so as to move forward into the new. For healing to occur, you have to be willing to move beyond the comfort zone and to face your fears and explore the unknown. By risking, we expand our boundaries and then in some strange and miraculous way, spirit finds a way to come in and support us. We may be sent the right person at the right time or something totally unexpected may suddenly appear or the next step becomes apparent.

In working with disease, illness or any imbalance, we have to treat the whole person not just disease otherwise it becomes a fragmented approach, like trying to patch up parts that don't work properly. Healing creates a synthesis between the mind, body and spirit. In Esoteric healing, disease is seen as discord in the soul and mind, and that when there is inner dissatisfaction this will be reflected outwardly. Although many doctors now recognize that illnesses have a psychosomatic aspect, they still do not really understood how deep the connection is between the thoughts and feelings and their effect on the physical body. Although both the fields of medicine and psychology have progressed tremendously, they are still miles apart. Ayurveda links the two by embracing both the medical aspect of health and the esoteric and offers healing modalities and techniques that diminish the boundaries and create an awareness of the union that is possible between the mind, body and spirit.

To create a new body, a body of bliss that is vital, radiant and energetic, we need to first deprogramme, to gradually erase the old programme and replace it with a new one. This takes consistent awareness and effort so as not to slip back into old habits and old ways of thinking. If for example someone has an addiction, it is not enough to just take away the substance they are addicted to, you have to find out what lies behind the addiction, what is the cause of the distress that makes the person want to reach for this particular substance. They know that what they are doing is harmful for their body but they go unconscious because they want the quick fix and are not ready to look at what lies behind the addiction. There is an underlying intelligence in the body; a knowingness that can be accessed and that can restore balance, peace and harmony within. The best way to access this intelligence is through meditation.

It is not your outer appearance that is important but who you are inside and how you feel. Bliss is an inner experience; it is more than just a moment of fleeting happiness or joy, it is an ongoing state, which leads to what the mystics call samadhi. When one is full of bliss, it radiates outwards and has a magnetizing effect. When we tap into the constant, pulsating reservoir of life force energy and feel it flowing abundantly through the body, then we truly know what it means to be fully alive. This is bliss consciousness, which is the essence of real spiritual work. As we get glimpses into bliss consciousness, we start to see the deeper meaning of life, the connectedness of all things and that nothing is by chance.

One of the most important aspects in healing is the work of the heart, opening the heart chakra and healing the wounds of the heart. By releasing the emotional pain from the past that gets locked in the body and especially in the area of the heart, we can free ourselves to experience deeper levels of love, ecstasy and bliss. When someone hurts us, we tend to contract and close down. The challenge is to stay open and go deeply into the experience until it is fully integrated and then move on. In this way, we can deal with it consciously and get a clearer perspective and move beyond it instead of suppressing, ignoring and holding onto to it, which creates unfinished business. When the connection between the heart and mind is open and the energy flows unrestricted between the two, then gradually all the other chakras come into balance and we regain our power and strength.

Love energy is the most potent and powerful force in the universe; it can dissolve barriers and create breakthroughs. If there were more love in the world towards our fellow human beings, the world would not be in the state it is in today. The vibration of love is the highest of vibrations and has the ability to heal. Jesus was the greatest healer ever known and he used the power of love. Mothers know how to soothe their children and heal their pain simply through love.

Our aura, the light energy field around the body reflects our vibrational level. When the body is sick, it emanates a certain vibration; we have to transform the sick vibrations. Hands on healers transmit healing energy to a person who is ill or in pain with the intention of clearing and lifting the vibration of the body so that it can heal itself. The body will use the healing energy in whatever way it can; the energy will go where it is most needed not necessarily to the problem you are trying to heal. We have to become aware of the vibrations we give out, for what we give out is what we will receive, like attracts like. By becoming sensitive to different vibrational fields, we can choose to avoid negative people, situations and places.

A question that always comes up around healing, is why do some people heal and others don't. There are many factors involved in the healing process, including karmic issues, which are difficult to understand. Sometimes there is an unconscious resistance to healing, for some reason a person does not want to heal, they want to maintain the situation because they are not ready for change or to forgive or let go. Their illness may provide a comfort zone, it is what they know and it may give them the attention or love they need or in some way bring meaning to their life. And sometimes we just don't know the answers and have to accept that some things are mysterious and unexplainable and beyond our comprehension. And as we look deeper, we find there is always a deeper meaning and many lessons, which need to be learnt.

In healing sessions something always happens, there is always an exchange of some sort, the results of which may not be visible to the physical eyes. It can also sometimes depend upon the skills and expertise of the healer. For healing to occur, there are many factors, which need to be addressed, healing is not about a quick fix. We may need to release something from the past, anger, resentment, judgment or fear and to learn how to accept, nourish and love ourselves.

If we don't make the necessary inner changes, the same illness may be recreated and that is why often a disease reoccurs or shows up again in another area or another form because the underlying patterns or problem has not been properly dealt with. When someone says that an illness is incurable, what they mean is that they don't know what to do, it is beyond their realm of expertise. Many people often go to healers after they have explored all the options, which the medical profession have to offer. Miracles do occur, with faith and trust in God or a higher power, all things are possible. As long as there is still breath in the body, there is always hope.

You can ask others to assist you in your healing process and it is good to get support but you also need to take an active role in your own healing process and become aware of what you can do for yourself. Ultimately when you learn to follow your intuition, you will know what is the best for you, trust your intuition and if something doesn't feel right don't do it. Visualization and meditation are tools to help open and empower you in your healing process.

In olden times, initiates of esoteric healing often lead a secluded life or lived in the temples. They were not allowed to practise healing until they had been through a rigorous training and achieved purification on many levels. The purity of a person and the development of their consciousness were considered essential parts of the training. When I did my Ayurvedic training, only those who practised specific advanced techniques of meditation were allowed to participate in the training. Meditation and Yoga were seen as important daily aspects of the training. In Tibet, doctors train for seven years but they also have to attain a high level of spiritual practice and perfect their meditation skills at the same time in order to qualify in Tibetan medicine.

Ayurveda and other schools of health, which focus on healing through natural means, try to avoid anything, which might be considered as invasive or violent to the body. For example operations are seen as a last resort in Chinese and Tibetan medicine, and avoided unless the situation is life threatening. They prefer not to cut out an organ or part of the body that is sick or diseased, but instead to try to save that part and find the root cause in order to heal it. Detoxification procedures or herbal medicine or other therapies may be used instead. Operations interfere with the energy flow, nerves, meridians and nadis are cut and this disturbs the energy system. It is advisable after any accident, trauma or operation to have healing or energywork to reconnect and rebalance the energetic flow.

The role of the healer is twofold, to help release the blocks within the patient so that the natural healing power can flow through unheeded and heal and also to act as a channel to bring in the divine energy, which will activate and accelerate the healing Often people come for healing because of a physical problem or an emotional crisis. If they are open, this usually leads them to a deeper exploration into themselves and the desire to know more. Through healing we can uncover many hidden facets of ourselves, parts that were hidden away or suppressed will slowly be drawn to the surface. There is a natural desire towards integration and wholeness.

Healing is a vast subject and sometimes healing can come in unexpected ways. Every culture has something to offer to the field of healing, there is so much to learn. Deep loving relationships and tender care are healing and emotional support plays an important part in the process. Breathing practises and meditation are major keys in healing and take us beyond the limitations of the mind. Unexpected miracles happen every day, healing belongs to the field of the unexplainable and the miraculous.

In Esoteric healing several factors are said to lie at the root of most illnesses and imbalances. It is believed that each soul has a specific destiny and life purpose and certain soul lessons. These are related to qualities and attributes that a person needs to develop to expand their consciousness. Inhibited soul life through the inability to express one's real self or to fulfil one's life purpose or the inability to flow with life in a natural way, result in a feeling of suppression, congestion, resentment or stuckness. In order to release these blockages and receive healing on a deep cellular level, it is thought that the person needs to embrace the spiritual as well and that this can lead to a more meaningful, higher quality of life.

You have to take full responsibility for your choices and what you create and not blame others for your circumstances but instead to look for solutions. Karmic issues from other lives may also influence your present situation, sometimes it is difficult to see the whole picture but as you work on your present issues, you can also clear the patterns of the past, which are related.

Transforming emotional discord and negativity will purify your vibrational field, which is affected by everything you think, feel and do. As you change, the vibrations you give out will change too and then you will attract different circumstances into your life. You need to detoxify the physical body, but you also need to detoxify mentally and emotionally as well. If you are stressed or angry or resentful this will recreate the same situations again and again. In order for transformation to take place at a cellular level there has to be a desire to change one's self and to live a life of integrity through not being afraid to speak and live one's truth. By engaging in transformational work and embracing the spiritual path and being of service to humanity, the karmic scales can be balanced.

Illness is the result of blocked energy, wrong attitudes, negative influences, emotional discord, mistreating or neglecting the body, overindulgence, addictive behaviour, destructive habits or karmic influences This results in a breakdown in the energy system, nervous system or the immune system and consequently affects every other organ and system in the body. There is a deep correlation between inner attitudes and outer circumstances, which is known as cause and effect. Through the study of cause and effect and the related circumstances, we are able to gain more insight and to see the truth. Gradually with time, an unveiling can occur that permits us to see more clearly how certain situations were created and what needs to be done to rectify them. As you begin to see the correlations and interconnectedness of all things, people and events, you start to get a sense of the larger picture.

"With God all things are possible." Faith in a divine source or higher power that is far greater than the ordinary human being is an important component of healing. Prayer and meditation can connect us to this source so that grace, assistance and healing can be given. Having a regular spiritual practice is an important part of any holistic approach. If you want to create a body of bliss, you have to understand what it means to live in a blissful state and reprogramme the cells with bliss consciousness. Energy follows thought and thought creates reality. Never underestimate the power of the mind and its ability to heal or the power of divine assistance. The potential for healing and transformation is always there. As the bones are the physical basis of the body and the immune system is the physical support system of the body, so trust, love, inner peace and harmony are the basis of spiritual development and healing.

8 - ENERGYWORK, ENHANCING THE VITAL LIFE FORCE

As we explore deeper into health and healing, we can move beyond the purely physical, to the energy level. As well as a physical body, we also have a more subtle body known as the energy body. Many people are not aware of their energy body and don't realize it exists simply because they cannot see it. Only those who are clairvoyant or who have developed extra sensory perception can see energy, but most people can feel the movement of energy once they become more sensitive. Energy work is considered to be the core of true healing in many traditions and especially in the exploration into consciousness and self-development. Energywork is a complicated science that includes knowledge of the energy body, the aura, which is the energy field that surrounds the body, the chakras, the major and minor energy centres and the nadis, the energy channels, which link everything together. When you work on an energy level, you can influence the physical, the mental and the emotional.

Most of the information that is available on energywork has filtered through to the West from the Yogis in India and the Lamas in Tibet. They are masters in this field and their whole life's work is primarily dedicated to the investigation of consciousness and energy. It takes many years of deep study to understand the workings of the energy system. In esoteric healing, it is believed that all disease starts with a loss of energy created by an imbalance or blockage in the energy system, which is related to many factors including emotional discord and disharmony, which affects the physical body and manifests as disease. When someone has a strong energy body and a good energy flow, they will also have a strong immune system and not be affected by outer circumstances or imbalances.

From the yogic point of view, how the life force energy flows is one of the most important aspects of health and is a reflection of everything that is happening in the body. If the energy flows well, the body will be able to cleanse, heal and rebalance all the systems of the body including strengthening the immune system. Where there is an insufficient flow of energy or blocks in the energy flow, this will result in low vitality, poor health and toxicity, which may lead to further congestion, restriction and disease.

The energy body consists of major and minor energy centres called chakras and marmas, which are junction points that are located at specific parts of the body. There is also a complex network of 350.000 nadis which link up the marmas and chakras. Prana, the vital life force flows through these tiny channels. The three major energy channels that flow through the spine are called Shushuma, Ida and Pingola.

When prana is abundant and flows unheeded throughout the body, we feel dynamically alive, strong and empowered, mentally alert and creative and have a limitless source of energy. When the energy flow is interrupted, blocked or constricted in any area, then the corresponding organs become weak and dysfunctional and this can lead to disease. Interferences in the energy flow can be created through many different factors including stress, trauma, negativity, emotional crisis, depression, fear, anger, lethargy, accidents, operations and toxicity. Other factors, which can contribute to disruptions in the energy flow, are overworking, lack of exercise, incorrect diet, overeating, smoking, drugs, antibiotics, sleeping tablets and tranquillisers. It is usually a combination of factors, which create an imbalance that has been manifesting in the body over a period of time.

When the energy level is low, the immune system becomes weakened and this makes us more vulnerable to disease. A disruption usually occurs first on an energy level and then a physical imbalance or discomfort may appear. Over the years as the imbalances increase and if they are not corrected, a breakdown in one of the systems may occur. Imbalances need to be corrected on an energy level and through a change of lifestyle factors, which produced them in the first place.

There are seven major energy centres in the body called chakras. The chakras are powerful energy vortexes that govern the 7 ductless glands in the body, which constitute the endocrine system. The endocrine glands regulate all the body functions including metabolism and the process of ageing. When any one gland is out of balance this will affect the other glands and create an imbalance in the corresponding energy centre and a disruption in the energy flow. When all the energy centres work efficiently together and the energy flows abundantly throughout the body, then all the organs and systems of the body will work harmoniously together as nature intended, and healing and regeneration can naturally take place.

Balancing the energy system is considered important in all natural systems of healing. Balance is the key. When the energy system of the body is balanced and all the physical body systems work efficiently together, then harmony and radiant health result. There is an important connection between the energy system and the endocrine system (hormonal flow) and between the energy system and the nervous system. They are very closely linked and affect each other. Stress and emotional discord affect the energy body and upset hormonal balance, which then causes physical problems.

Everything that we think, feel and do affects our energy body, either positively or negatively. Every thought, word and experience is registered within the energy body. When there is a build up of emotional turmoil or distress in the energy body, it needs to be discharged; otherwise this will create an energy blockage, which can then manifest as a corresponding physical blockage. This will be seen in more detail in the chapter on chakras, which explains the connection between the different chakras, glands and different parts of the body. Suppressed emotions and emotional turmoil are the root cause of many diseases.

The energy system feeds and provides the fuel for the whole body including all the organs and different systems. Once you understand the interrelatedness of the different systems of the body and the energy body and how they work together, then you will realize how important it is to maintain good energy levels and not to drain or strain oneself. Strain on any one system can impair its proper functioning and this will create pressure on the other systems as they try to take the weight off the one that is not functioning efficiently. This is very evident in the case of stress. With a continuous build up of stress, eventually a breaking point is reached, in one person this could show up as a nervous breakdown or extreme tiredness which results in the inability to work or function properly. In another it could be a stomach ulcer, heart problem, cancer or immune related disease.

Tension, anger, frustration, fear or dissatisfaction get locked into the body, tighten the muscles and irritate the nervous system, this results in an energetic imbalance. Every crisis and trauma is registered somewhere in the body, in the cells, the tissues, the muscles and the bones. These destructive emotions need to be released otherwise they act like poison in the body. When poison stays in the body for too long, it spreads and causes disease. Energywork, rebirthing, pranayamas, chanting, Yoga, dance, movement, psychotherapy and other means of self-expression are all ways to release the tension and holding and can open us to new levels of expression and freedom.

If the vital energy centres function too slowly then there will be a deterioration of the body and premature ageing will take place. If the energy centres function too fast and too much energy is used up there will be exhaustion and burn out. When there is not enough energy or it is blocked for some reason, we start to draw on our energy reserves. The body has the necessary reserves to accommodate overload for a certain period of time, but if we live off those reserves for too long, they will be depleted and then nothing will be left and a breakdown will occur. It is imperative to take enough time to rest and regenerate and to recharge our batteries on a daily basis.

Some people think they have an inexhaustible source of energy, and keep stretching themselves to the limit, rushing about never having a peaceful moment but eventually this takes its toll on their health. Excessive tiredness and nervous exhaustion, eventually lead to burn out. Women often feel this when they reach menopause. At a time when they need to remain balanced and draw on their energy reserves, unexpectedly they may discover that their reserves are empty. Getting enough deep rest, relaxation, meditation and quiet time are absolutely essential for everyone but even more so for working mothers who have many demands placed upon them. It is not easy to maintain the balance between working, looking after a home and children and looking after oneself.

The role of the modern woman has changed and everyone in the family needs to help and pull their weight in taking responsibility for the household, including the children. Busy women, especially working women often feel guilty about taking time for themselves, they feel they ought to be able to cope and do all the things they would do if they had more time at home. Women have a more delicate nervous system than men and they have to learn how to take care of it in the right way. If you feel stretched, on overload or exhausted, it is essential for your health and well-being that you find some time every day for yourself to centre and be quiet in order to recuperate and re-energize yourself, this is not a luxury, it is a necessity. A daily meditation and a weekly energy balancing, healing or reflexology session can be lifesavers in the midst of a busy and active lifestyle.

To understand the energy body, you have to think in terms of energy. The easiest way to do that is to become aware of your own energy levels. How do you experience your energy? Do you feel you have enough energy to do all the things you would like to do? Do you wake up feeling good and bouncing with energy or do you feel slow or sluggish in the morning, does it take you some time to get going? Can you go through the day without getting tired or by the afternoon do you feel depleted? Is this depletion ongoing or just sometimes. Are you aware of why your energy is low at these times? Does this happen at certain times of the day or the month or during certain seasons, is there a cycle to these ups and downs and are you aware of what affects it? Do you feel low in energy during the change of season?

How does your menstruation affect you, do you feel tired before or during menstruation?

The lunar cycle affects most people even if they are not consciously aware of it. Some people are at their best during the days of the full moon cycle, and have lots of energy and feel creative. Other people feel pressure from the full moon and are easily irritated or don't sleep well at that time. There are more accidents and suicides around the three day cycle of the full moon than during the rest of the month. During new moon, the energy is lower, for the moon is in a resting phase. You may find that your energy is lower too at this time; you make not feel so creative and may need to rest more, so it is best not to plan too many activities around the time of new moon.

Start monitoring your energy and notice how you feel energetically through different times of the day. Observe what things lift your energy and make you feel good, also what things drain your energy, including people, places, foods and drinks. Some people are energy drainers, they just take and take and leave you feeling drained, avoid being with such people especially if you are feeling low. Start tracking your energy, watch your energy cycles, be aware of how they fluctuate and what affects them.

Lack of energy comes from living an unbalanced or stressful lifestyle. This occurs through not paying proper attention to your needs and not listening to your body and slowing down when you need to. Ingesting toxic substances, not eating a balanced diet, eating too much and not getting enough exercise or fresh air will make you feel heavy and lethargic and block your energy flow. Do things that make you feel good and put new healthy habits into practice that will increase your energy level.

We have huge resources of untapped energy within us, just waiting to be released. As you release stagnant, blocked energy, you will feel so much better, more vibrant and alive Yoga, breathwork, meditation, rebirthing, energy balancing and acupuncture are some of the most effective ways to release blocked energy. When you look

163

around, how many people do you see who look fresh and radiant and are full of energy? As people get older most of them lose their vitality and sparkle, this is not because of their age, but because of their lifestyles, incorrect diet, too much stress and negative thoughts and feelings. You can be vibrant, energetic and youthful at any age providing you take good care of yourself and have a positive attitude towards life. In India there are many Yoga teachers in their eighties or nineties who are an inspiration, they are vibrant and full of energy, they know how to master their energy.

Increasing your energy level starts with self-awareness. By observing your daily routine and lifestyle habits, you can discover what affects you energetically and make the necessary changes in your life that will make you feel so much better. Deep down, most people already know what would really benefit them; they have an intuitive sense of what they need. This is where meditation is so helpful, it brings you closer to the real self and makes you aware of what is really right for you and naturally points you in the direction of more sattvic and joyful living.

Rio guarana is a herb from the Amazon, which was mentioned before in the herbal section, it is a food supplement, a natural energizer and a general tonic. It boosts the energy in a natural way. It can be taken on going or just when you need it and it has no side effects. It is very helpful when you are under pressure or tired or low in energy, also around the time of menstruation, during menopause or times of transition. It is best taken first thing in the morning on an empty stomach. Make sure to buy the pure Rio guarana seed and not an extract or guarana mixed with other herbs which would give only a minimal effect.

When guarana was first brought to the West, it was used primarily by acupuncturists who discovered that guarana released energy blocks and that its tonic effect increased both mental and physical energy. They also found it relieved pain. Measuring the energy flow in the various meridians with the Vega test instrument indicated a definite change in the twelve meridians and showed that blocked energy is undoubtedly released after taking guarana. The Amazonian natives have long known the secret of guarana and its energizing properties and take it daily, especially when going on long treks through the Amazon.

When our energy is blocked, it can affect us in various ways, we may feel physically or emotionally low, or lack enthusiasm for life, which can result in depression. With our modern day lifestyles, there is a tendency to sit too much, eat too much and not exercise enough, this stagnates us both physically and energetically. A stagnant lifestyle causes premature ageing. Walking every day improves the circulation, is good for the heart and gets the energy moving. Yoga is one of the best practises to release energy blocks and improve energy flow. A daily workout of yoga postures combined with pranayama breathing will improve flexibility by opening up the body and activating the vital energy centres. This will enable the prana, the life force, to move through the body, energize the brain and to create better coherence between the mind and the body. It will also stimulate agni, the digestive fire in the solar plexus, thereby increasing detoxification of the body and improving metabolism and the assimilation of nutrients.

As blocked energy is released, a surge of energy may be felt moving through the body, or little ripples or pulsations of energy. Intense heat in certain parts of the body is also a sign of energy been activated, this is often felt in meditation or during Yoga. At the bottom of the spine, lies the kundalini energy; in ancient texts this has been pictured as a coiled serpent or snake. In most people the kundalini energy remains dormant and never rises, so they never feel the full force of the powerful energy that lies sleeping within them. Anyone who has experienced a kundalini awakening knows it to be the most powerful of experiences, beyond description, like a tremendous force rushing at great speed throughout the body, followed by the feeling of deep cleansing, opening and bliss. Awakening the kundalini force is associated with enlightenment. The kundalini energy is considered to be the ultimate source of sustenance, which shatters all illusions and opens the person to higher states of consciousness. Kundalini awakening takes years of spiritual practise and should not be attempted without the guided expertise of an experienced teacher. Clearing of samskaras, ill deeds of the past have to be removed first.

The pure life force energy that flows through and around the body is called prana. Prana is everywhere, and has been called the Divine Nectar, the ultimate healing power. Prana comes from the very source of life. Yogis have studied prana and learnt to master its flow, both by drawing it into the body and increasing its flow throughout the body. Prana is mysterious; it is the essence that maintains life. Through refining our senses and developing our sensitivity, we can become more aware of prana. We can observe where it flows and where it doesn't. The more we learn about prana, the deeper we come to know ourselves, the workings of the universe and the divine source of all life.

We take prana into the body through outer resources, through the breath; through the skin and through the nourishment we take into our bodies. The sun is one of the most potent life giving forces available to us, it sustains all of nature and mankind. If you take a few minutes a day to connect to the sun energy, you will feel enlivened and stimulated. If you live in a climate that permits it, practising pranayamas and Yoga postures outside whilst facing the sun and feeling the rays of the sun upon your body has a cleansing and healing effect. The Essenes knew the power of sun energy and it was an important part of their healing programme. They called upon the Angel of the Sun to nourish their mind and bodies and accelerate healing. Sun worshipping has been known through the ages. There is a limitless amount of energy in the universe, which we can utilize, but we have to learn how to access and assimilate it rather than using up our own energy reserves.

Sun energized water is very therapeutic and cleansing. If you put a glass jug of fresh water out in the sun for five to ten minutes, the sun energy will activate it. You can also add a clear, clean, quartz crystal to the water to accelerate the vibrations. We can energize our foods by putting them in the sun for a few minutes. Freezing food has exactly the opposite effect, it kills the food. Kirlian experiments show that frozen food is dead food and contains no life force energy at all.

Fresh air, especially mountain air or sea air contains a lot of prana, you can feel it, you breathe it in and it feels good. Try to go out into nature as often as possible so you can absorb the prana, or if you live in a city then go to a park where there are lots of trees. Leaning against a tree, will give you extra energy, when you feel low find a big, strong, old tree and lean against it and feel its energy. Walking on the earth or the beach barefoot helps you get grounded and you can draw up the earth energy through the soles of the feet. Try to walk barefoot as often as possible, it stimulates the nerve endings in the soles of the feet. If you lie down on the ground and connect to Mother Earth, you can release all the tension from your body down into the ground and then draw up the earth energy to replenish you.

There are many natural, sattvic foods, minerals and herbs, which give you prana, especially those that are eaten in their natural state. Fruit is one of the most highly pranic foods you can eat. Review the superfoods list and sattvic foods to see which foods will give you the most energy and avoid those, which make you feel dull and lifeless.

Ayurvedic medicine, has long known the secret of balancing prana between different parts of the body, disturbances in prana can be felt in the pulse. It is said, that when the body is truly healthy, prana flows through the body like a gushing river, cleansing, purifying, enlivening and nourishing. The power of prana determines the strength or weakness of the body. In a weak or sick body, the life force will be weak. Emphasis is therefore placed upon observing the life force energy in the body and becoming aware of what affects it, weakens, drains or impedes its circulation.

There is no better or more powerful way to recharge the energy on a daily basis than through meditation. In meditation, prana can be received directly from the source. The cosmic energy is limitless in its supply and this is what healers align with in order to act as channels and draw in the cosmic energy and pass it on to those who need it. You can do this yourself through aligning with the cosmic energy in meditation to lift your own energy levels and to heal imbalances or disease. This is the real source of abundance, which never runs out. How much energy a healer or individual is able to access and draw upon, depends upon the consciousness and self-development of the person. Many healers who are not properly aligned and do not have enough knowledge of working with energy, actually use their own energy and this eventually leads to burn out.

Energy medicine is the true source of healing and hopefully one day in the near future, it will be better understood and more people will seek this way of healing. As your senses become more refined and your sensitivity increases, you will be able to feel more intensely what is happening in a healing session and become more conscious of what sort of treatment is right for you. Be selective and don't just let anyone work on you, get a sense of their energy and how conscious the person appears to be and whether you get a good feeling from them. By looking at things in terms of energy, many things will become clearer and you will see some of the changes that you need to make, always let your intuition, your inner knowingness guide you. Everything begins with awareness and when you start to put your attention on increasing your energy level, your intuition will guide you step by step on what to do.

One of the main functions of Yoga asanas (postures) is to clear physical, emotional and energy blocks in the body so that the energy can flow more freely and then healing can take place. In India, in many yoga centres, physical illnesses are healed purely through the practise of yoga asanas, pranayamas and meditation. Once this has been achieved, the body can then activate the powerful kundalini energy within and receive more energy from higher sources, but first the blocks have to be removed.

There is a close connection between energywork and breathwork. Pranayamas are special Yogic breathing techniques that activate the brain and help circulate the prana throughout the body. Pranayamas

168

are usually practised before meditation. There are different pranayamas to activate different parts of the body. Alternative nostril breathing quietens the mind, increases oxygen flow to the brain and improves co-ordination between the left and right sides of the brain. It can also be practised before sleeping to induce a more relaxed state during sleep. There are pranayamas to cleanse and release deep tension in the abdomen and to heal and energize each organ.

Around the physical body, is an energy field known as the aura. The aura reflects and mirrors what is happening in the body. Many imbalances first show up in the auric field before manifesting as disease in the body. The aura is visible to those with psychic abilities and can also be photographed by Kirlian photography. Everything is registered in the aura; the colours of the aura reflect one's physical health, mental attitudes, and spiritual development. No two people have the same aura. Sometimes you may not be able to see a person's aura but you may sense it. We can often sense a person's energy, it may feel good and we feel drawn to them or we may feel repelled or fearful, something tells us to stay away. People who take a lot of drugs have an erratic energy or there may be an auric dark cloud around the head area because the drugs have affected the brain. On the other hand, saints are depicted with a white or yellow aura around their heads; this reflects their spiritual development.

Whether we are sick or healthy, filled with energy or depleted, this will show up in our aura. By brushing your aura every day you can create a sense of calm especially to areas where there is pain. It is the same gentle movement you would do if you were stroking a cat but you don't actually touch the body, you keep your hand about two centimetres away from the body and gently brush the aura. You can also relax, listen to soothing music and place your hands on parts of your body that need healing.

Our energy is our life source, the life sustaining link between us and the universe. When we think 'in terms of radiant health and vitality, we must also think in terms of abundant energy. No matter what age you are, if the life force energy flows through you abundantly and freely, you will be able to enjoy life to the full because you will never feel drained or tired, and you will awaken every day feeling happy and ready for what the day may bring.

9 - THE CHAKRAS

There are seven main vortexes of energy in the body called chakras. Each of these chakras corresponds to a certain area of the body and is related to a particular gland and organs. The chakras are located internally along the spine and when they function effectively, they radiate out energy from both the front and back of the body. Although the chakras are not physical centres, their movement can be felt by those who are sensitive. Heat may sometimes be experienced in a chakra, as it is being activated or energized.

The first chakra known as the base chakra is located at the bottom of the spine, between the coccyx and the pubic bone. The second chakra, the sacral chakra is located in the lower abdomen below the navel, the third is the solar plexus, between the diaphragm and the navel, the fourth is the heart chakra, in the centre of the chest, the fifth is the throat chakra in the pit of the throat, the sixth chakra known as the ajna centre or the third eye is located at the level of the forehead in the centre of the brain. The seventh chakra, the crown chakra is on the crown of the head. In some systems they recognize an eighth chakra that is located in the spleen on the left side of the abdomen, but most systems incorporate the spleen chakra with the solar plexus.

Understanding the function and working with the chakras is a deep science, which takes many years of study, contemplation and meditation. Through the chakras we can receive cosmic energy and activate healing and transform the energy level of the body. When any one chakra or associated gland is not functioning properly, it will affect the other chakras and glands. The whole energy system needs to be well balanced and to work harmoniously so as to create a good energy flow. Any dysfunction on the level of the chakras and the energy system affects the corresponding glands and will eventually manifest as an imbalance or disruption on the physical level.

When working in the field of healing, either for one's self or for others, some basic knowledge of the chakras is useful as it gives insights into the mind-body connection and the physical and non physical realities, how closely they are linked and the way they affect each other. In esoteric schools the chakras are also called the seven seals, the seven doorways and the seven initiations, they are the gateways to higher self-development and knowledge. When fully awakened they have also been called the seven blazing suns.

The study of the chakras is complex, many yogis and advanced spiritual teachers spend a lifetime learning and deepening their knowledge of the chakra system. The chakras reflect the health, well-being and spiritual development of the individual. Some systems differ slightly in their opinion as to which organs are aligned with each chakra but the overall working of the chakra system is fundamentally the same.

Each chakra lies at the centre of a vast network of nadis, tiny energy channels, which form the energy body, also known as the vital body or the subtle body. The chakras receive, transform and distribute the life force energy. When they work efficiently together, they are able to send energy throughout the body and clear any blockages. However if the chakras or channels are blocked, congested or contracted, then the life force energy cannot flow freely and this leads to imbalances, weakening and degeneration of different bodily systems and organs. Mastering the energy system and lifting the vibrational energy level of the body is imperative for regeneration to take place. Becoming more relaxed and developing a state of inner peace and harmony, helps recreate balance and healing in the energy system. The chakras are subtle, sensory organs, which register everything, comprehending the function of the chakras is very subtle work.

Because of the stress and strain of every day life and the challenges that most of us have to face, it is not always easy to maintain emotional equilibrium and this is where we need to be constantly alert. By recharging ourselves with energy through meditation, pranayamas or other practises on a daily basis, we can also release or transform any negative energy that we may have received and retained in the body. If your vital energy is depleted, the physical resistance will be lowered and you may feel more vulnerable or emotional. A constant state of stress and irritation, hyperactivity or anger agitates the nervous system and this affects the energy system and creates problems on the physical level. The body is very resilient but constant emotional discord and stressful ways of living wear it out prematurely.

As mentioned before, each of the chakras is related to certain parts of the body and to specific glands and organs. So you can imagine that the body is divided into seven sections and each section is governed by one of the chakras. At the same time we have to hold the holistic viewpoint and remember that everything is interrelated and that for total health and complete balance, all the chakras, glands and organs need to function harmoniously together. Imbalances or diseases in a particular area indicate which chakra is imbalanced. Understanding the chakras helps us to recognize what lies behind imbalances and disease and how emotional discord effects the mind and the body.

Following is an outline of each chakra, its functions and correlations and the problems that can occur in relation to each chakra.

The First Chakra

The first chakra is known as the base or root chakra. It is situated at the coccyx, at the bottom of the spine, between the pubic bone and the anus. There is an important connection between the base chakra and the crown chakra on the top of the head. When we meditate, we can draw energy into the body through the crown chakra and bring it all the way down the spine to the base chakra. We can send energy down into the earth from the base chakra in order to ground, stabilize and draw energy up from the earth into the body. When the base chakra functions well, we feel present, stable and secure in the world.

If we develop the upper centres but are not in touch with the first chakra, we may feel spacey and be unrealistic.

The base chakra is the foundation of the physical body and is related to the spinal column. It is the support system of the body and supports all the other chakras. How you sit and stand affects your whole body especially the spine and your energy. Keeping your spine straight whilst sitting or standing is important. It is not by coincidence that yogis and advanced meditators sit in the lotus position to meditate, this creates a physical support for the body whilst drawing down the higher energies as well as enabling the energy to flow up and down the spine freely without any postural obstruction. It takes practice and time to be able to sit in the lotus posture, Hatha Yoga gradually prepares the body for this.

The base of the spine houses the kundalini, the dynamic, primal energy force of the body, which when activated moves upwards through the three main energy channels known as Sushumma, Ida and Pingala. The kundalini is the most powerful healing force that can awaken a person to higher states of consciousness that bring complete clarity, deeper insights into life as well as releasing tremendous energy, strength and power. Before the kundalini can be awakened and activated, purification needs to take place on all levels.

The base chakra is related to the adrenal glands, which are located immediately above the kidneys. They produce 50 different hormones, one of the most important being adrenaline, which creates the fight or flight response. The base chakra is also associated with the bones, teeth, nails, legs, bladder, rectum and the immune system. If our base, our support system is weak, then the immune system will be affected and weaken too. There is an important connection between the base chakra and the kidneys. Some systems say the kidneys are governed by the third chakra because of their location, others say that because the kidneys are linked through the ureters to the bladder that they are governed by the base chakra, both are essentially correct. For the purpose of healing, I prefer to classify the kidneys within the region of the third chakra.

The first chakra has to do with issues of security and survival, also about setting boundaries. If you feel secure, safe and comfortable in the world, then your support system, both physical and emotional will be strong. If you feel unsupported and alone or worry a lot this can result in lower back pain, constipation, overweight and other problems in this area. Resentment affects the bones, as does holding onto the past and being unable to let go or to forgive.

The first chakra can be activated through paying attention to your posture and how you stand and sit and grounding yourself well and feeling that you are fully in your body. When you walk, feel the connection between your feet and the earth and draw the energy all the way down to your feet. Try to spend time regularly in nature, watch the sunrise and sunset and connect with Mother Earth, this helps with the grounding process.

Reflexology and the Metamorphic technique help activate all the chakras by working on the corresponding points and by stimulating all the thousands of nerve endings in the feet. By having your feet worked on or massaged regularly, you become more aware of your feet and legs and this helps with grounding.

The Yoga postures which specifically help open the base chakra are sitting cross legged in lotus or half lotus position, sitting with the knees up and the soles of the feet together and the bridge posture (lifting up the middle part of the body).

The base chakra is associated with the colour red. If you feel drawn to the colour red then wear it or use the colour red in the house. Red is associated with vitality and awakening the life force, you can visualize the base chakra as red during meditation. Eating foods of the same colour as the chakra, are said to have a stimulating and balancing effect on that particular chakra. Some red foods are tomatoes, red peppers, red apples, beets, red cabbage, aubergines and radish.

The Second Chakra

The second chakra is known as the sacral chakra and is located within the pelvic girdle. It is related to the ovaries and governs the reproductive system, reproductive organs, the hips, pelvis and the intestinal area. It is linked with the kidneys and the bladder. The second chakra has to do with all sexual and reproductive functions, regulation of the female hormone cycle, fertility, sensuality and nourishment. It is also where the creative energy is germinated. The ovaries produce oestrogen and progesterone, which are responsible for the development of female sexual characteristics, menstruation, pregnancy and menopause. Our emotional state deeply influences this area and this becomes more evident around the time before menstruation and during menopause. The second chakra is associated with the water element and all liquids in the body including the blood, the lymph, gastric juices and saliva. It is therefore important to drink approximately one litre of water a day to help purify the body and to do regular kidney cleansing.

Problems related to the second chakra include menstrual problems, infertility, vaginal infections, tumours and cancers of the female organs. These have to do with feelings of lack of self worth, not receiving enough nourishment and feeling unloved, also difficulties in giving or receiving love. The pelvis is often referred to as the real seat of shakti, the feminine power. When a woman is not in touch with her power or she gives it away to others especially to men, it is usually because she feels insecure about herself as a woman. If she is unsure of her sensuality or sexuality or doesn't feel good about her body, then this creates disharmony and may manifest as problems in the area of the second chakra. The problems may come from childhood or the parents' attitude towards the child or towards sexuality. If the child did not receive enough affection, tenderness or touching and hugging or there were male or female issues in the family, this may have created low self esteem. There may be guilt or suppressed feelings around sexuality, which get stored in this area. Issues to do with emotional eating and addictions and never having enough, stem from not having enough emotional nourishment especially during childhood.

The key to healing problems in this area, lies in learning to nourish one's self and not expecting others to do it for you. The sacral chakra is all about nourishing oneself. The baby in the womb receives nourishment from its mother. Do things that make you feel really good, pamper and treat yourself. Open yourself to new ideas especially in the area of self-development. Being receptive and opening to receive is associated with the second chakra. Nourishing yourself also has to do with living healthily, eating the right foods, getting enough sleep and rest and taking time for yourself.

Take a close look at your relationships and issues around intimacy and sexuality. Don't suppress your feelings or hold back, this creates blockages. Embrace the feminine shakti power that lies in the womb and give birth to a new, sacred woman.

The main Yoga posture to help open the sacral chakra is the cobra pose.

The sacral chakra is associated with the colour orange. Orange is stimulating and energizing. Eat orange foods such as oranges, mandarins, carrots, orange peppers, pumpkin and squash.

The Third Chakra

The third chakra known as the solar plexus chakra governs the whole abdominal area from the diaphragm to the navel. It is related to the pancreas gland and governs the stomach, liver, gall bladder, kidneys, spleen and the colon. In some systems of healing, the spleen is thought of as one of the most important organs. The pancreas gland produces insulin, which maintains the correct sugar level in the blood and glucagon, which raises the blood sugar level.

The solar plexus has to do with the functions of digestion, assimilation and metabolism, not only food but also digesting and assimilating life experiences. What is not digested or assimilated properly remains as a residue that can create a toxic layer. Eating disorders also have to do with issues that are related to the solar plexus. The digestive fire in the solar plexus, the agni, can purify physical toxins. When the solar plexus is overloaded either from overeating or too much stress resulting in over acidity, it becomes blocked and imbalanced. Constant worry, anxiety, fear and unresolved emotional issues affect the abdominal organs. Fear affects the kidneys and impedes circulation and anger poisons the liver. There is a connection between the eyes and the quality of our vision and what we see, both visually and intuitively. If the kidneys or liver are toxic, then the eyesight and our ability to have a greater vision of life may be affected. Frustration, anger and resentment cause stones in the liver, gall bladder and kidneys.

The third chakra is our power centre. Power is often misunderstood because it is so often abused. Power is very effective when it is used in the right way. Being empowered is about connecting to your true sense of self and acting on what feels right for you and having the strength and willpower to follow through on your intuition. When the third chakra is open, you feel empowered through an inner strength, which urges you to act and make the right decisions. When you know what you want and your priorities are clear, then you can assert yourself when necessary. Many women feel disempowered and are unable to assert themselves, they need to reclaim their power and look at what they are really afraid of.

There is a deep connection between loss of personal power and trust issues; there may be feelings of inadequacy or guilt or a fear of rejection. As a child, the unfolding personality may have been suppressed, overpowered, smothered or overprotected by the parents or later in life by a partner and this may have resulted in low self-esteem or a loss of a true sense of self.

The solar plexus is the area in the body for centering; breathing into the solar plexus area helps release tension and relaxes the abdominal area. The solar plexus is a major purification centre both physically and emotionally. Unresolved issues from the past may get knotted in this area and can create a disconnection or an interrupted energy flow between the heart centre and the solar plexus.

When the first three chakras function harmoniously together, we feel supported and nourished within ourselves and a sense of fulfilment develops as we use the creative energy to move towards wholeness.

Yellow is the colour associated with the solar plexus, it is the colour of the sun, glowing, radiant and vital. By visualizing the solar plexus filled with yellow and using the colour yellow in your life, you can empower yourself and bring more joy into your life.

The main Yoga posture for the solar plexus is the bow pose. Yellow foods to include in your diet are wheat, rice, oats, corn, nuts, seeds and yellow pulses. The herbs marigold and camomile are soothing for this area.

The Fourth Chakra

The fourth chakra is located in the middle of the chest. It is related to the thymus gland, which regulates growth and metabolism and strengthens immune function. The fourth chakra governs the heart and the circulatory system, the breasts, shoulders, arms and lungs and is closely linked with the nervous system. The thymus is located behind the breastbone and by tapping it every day it strengthens the immune system.

The fourth chakra is connected with the physical heart and the emotional heart and understanding things from the level of the heart. It has to do with developing love and compassion, empathy, sympathy, sincerity and emotional warmth, learning to be sensitive without being vulnerable and expressing forgiveness.

If the heart chakra is closed or blocked or there are suppressed or buried feelings, there will be a difficulty either in giving or receiving love and problems may develop in this area. Disappointment, grief, pain, rejection, defensiveness or coldness and indifference can cause the heart chakra to close. This may result in the feeling of isolation, desperation, depression or the need for constant stimulation. Emotional traumas create emotional and physical congestion and energy blocks. Rebirthing can open and release these suppressed emotions and bring about a new sense of freedom and open the person to love again.

Heart disease, heart attacks, high blood pressure, blocked arteries; asthma, lung problems, breast cancer and other problems of this area are related to an inability to express or receive love or from holding onto something from the past which may have caused grief or despair. Sometimes, this may be so deeply buried that neither the person nor those around them realize what is going on. They may be totally out of touch with their feelings and put on a happy, outer façade to the world. Nothing is ever just physical. No one really knows what is going on deep inside a person, There may be layers and layers of emotional discord and unfinished business from the past that need to be addressed but have been pushed down. The issues of the heart are delicate ones and compassionate counselling and rebirthing and healing can do wonders in helping a person to clear and release the past.

Love and compassion can transform all negative vibrations if a person is willing to open to them. Through releasing, clearing, forgiving and pulling the thorns out of the heart, we open to the potential of personal transformation and healing. By learning to love oneself and working with the vibration of love, amazing changes can occur. The healing of the heart is the greatest work one can do.

The colours green and pink are associated with the heart. Green is the colour for harmony, healing and peace and pink is the colour for awakening love, tenderness and compassion. Rose quartz crystals and green crystals are useful in the work of awakening the heart.

Green foods are said to be good for the heart, eat lots of nourishing green salads and green vegetables.

The main Yoga asana to stimulate the heart chakra is the camel pose.

The Fifth Chakra

The fifth chakra is the throat chakra, known as the communication centre. The fifth chakra is situated in the area of the pit of the throat and it is also linked with a smaller chakra at the back of the neck at the bottom of the brain. These two centres are often seen as one as they function closely together. The throat chakra is related to the thyroid gland, which is responsible for metabolism. The throat chakra governs the whole throat region including the vocal chords, the mouth, the jaw, the neck, the upper lobes of the lungs, the bronchial tubes and the ears.

The throat centre is connected to everything to do with communication and self-expression. When the throat chakra is clear, you can communicate your needs clearly without hesitation or feelings of limitation or guilt. This chakra also has to do with the ability to express your ideas, your creativity and your truth without fear of being misunderstood or rejected. Being able to do this comfortably shows true independence and personal freedom.

When the throat chakra is open, there is a free flow of energy between the heart and the mind, between one's thoughts and feelings and the expression of both. The throat chakra is the bridge between the head and the heart. If there is difficulty in communication, between you and others or between the mind and the body or the heart and the mind, then there may be a block in the throat chakra. In my work as a healer, I have noticed that almost all women have throat chakra problems, women in general are afraid to express their deepest truths or to ask for what they want because of fear of being rejected or not being loved for who they truly are. The inability to freely express and communicate what lies in the heart creates a feeling of being suppressed and stifled, this may create emotional instability, moodiness or depression because the deeper needs are not being fulfilled.

When you have developed a strong sense of inner security and stability and have learnt how to nourish and empower yourself, then the ability to express yourself honestly without fear will emerge. You need to be able to say no to the demands and expectations of others when they don't feel right or go against what you believe in. Women often feel guilty about saying no but it is important to find the balance between nourishing oneself and nourishing and giving to others.

Thyroid or throat problems, irritable cough, gum, teeth and jaw problems and tension headaches, pain at the back of the neck and upper shoulders all indicate difficulties or an imbalance in the throat chakra area. If you hold yourself back from expressing your true self or your power or creativity, there will always be a feeling of lack. You may try to fill this lack with outer things, but it never works. The tone of the voice and what is said or not said indicates what is going on deep inside. If the tone is sharp or high-pitched, it indicates nervousness or tension, whereas a coarse or business like voice shows a lack of connectedness to one's feelings. A stutter or shyness show a difficulty in communicating whereas someone who is over talkative and has an inability to listen to others may be covering up emotions and not willing to connect to deeper levels of themselves. A weak or raspy voice indicates a blockage in expression. Someone who shouts a lot or speaks very loudly has control issues. Listening to people's voices is interesting and can tell you a lot about them.

To clear the throat chakra of old stagnant energy, you have to release the fear of speaking your truth and being yourself, it has to come from the heart. Try to be aware of the difference when you speak from the heart or from the mind. That is one of the benefits of counselling work; you can talk and speak your truth to someone who will listen to you compassionately with an open mind without judgement.

The colour light blue is associated with the throat chakra. Contemplate the light blue sky often, feel the soothing, calmness of a beautiful blue sky or wear the colour blue.

The Yoga postures for the throat chakra are the shoulderstand, the fish and neck exercises.

The Sixth Chakra

The sixth chakra is known as the Brow chakra, the Ajna centre or the centre of the third eye. The sixth chakra is associated with the pituitary gland, which is responsible for the chemistry of the body. It is considered to be the master gland, which orchestrates and oversees all the other glands. The sixth chakra governs the lower brain, the face, the left eye, the ears, nose, forehead and the central nervous system.

The main functions of the sixth chakra are related to developing both sides of the brain, the left and right side as well as opening the higher mental faculties. As the sixth chakra opens then the sixth sense starts to develop, which is related to the intuition, imagination, creative inspiration and psychic abilities. You may then start to experience intuitive flashes and receive deeper insights and find your creativity flows more easily. Geniuses and great masters in all fields including scientists, artists and musicians get their intuitive insights through the sixth chakra, some are more left brain oriented and others more right brained.

Problems in this area include brain tumours, blood clots in the head and brain, neurological disorders, blindness, deafness, migraine, headaches, tension, any nervous system related problems including anxiety, depression, and sleep disorders. Where there are eye and ear problems, there may be things we don't want to see or hear. The eyes are connected to the kidneys and liver and are affected by fear and anger. Confusion, scattered focus, the inability to concentrate or short or long-term memory difficulties are all sixth chakra related.

The sixth chakra is sometimes called the third eye because when it starts to open we see things differently; our consciousness starts to change and is influenced by the seventh chakra, which is associated with a higher, more spiritual vision of life. Then you gain more clarity and a new perspective, which wasn't there before and this can open you to new possibilities. You begin to understand the process of conscious creation and that you have the power to manifest your reality and that it is only your inhibitions or limitations that hold you back. By paying more attention to your sixth sense and listening and acting on your intuitive insights and creative ideas, you can change the quality of your life.

Most people have a tendency to be either left brain oriented or right brain oriented. Women tend to be more right brained although this does not mean that they do not also have a highly developed intellectual faculty too. In order to fully develop both our mental and intuitive powers, we need to develop both sides of our brain and engage in activities, which help us do this. The left-brain governs the intellectual, the pragmatic, the practical and the thinking aspects of life, whereas the right brain governs the intuitive, creative, artistic, sensitive and feeling side. If someone is very intellectual and the right side of the brain is not developed, they may lack feelings or be unable to express themselves well and dismiss the spiritual side of life. If someone is predominantly right brained but has not developed their left brain enough, they may have the tendency to be ungrounded or spaced out and have wonderful ideas but be unable to implement them or to organize their lives. Most of our schooling is left brained and for children who have more right brain tendencies this can create difficulties, not because they are not intelligent but because they function in a different way. From a young age, children need to be exposed to both and it is important to stimulate their imagination and creativity and not to ignore this faculty.

At any age, we must keep the mind active and stimulated through new challenges and activities and at the same time, develop peace of mind. Techniques of relaxation, meditation and visualization quieten the mind and give us the ability to access more expansive and unlimited states of mind.

The colours of indigo (dark blue) and purple are associated with the sixth chakra.

Alternate nostril breathing helps balance and activate both sides of the brain.

The Seventh Chakra

The seventh chakra is known as the crown chakra and is situated on the top of the head and governs the right eye and the upper part of the brain. It is associated with the pineal gland, which is located in the centre of the brain. The pineal gland produces melatonin at night especially during sleep and governs our body rhythms and cycles. When the production level of melatonin is low there is dullness and drowsiness in the brain and the ageing process is accelerated. Low melatonin levels can also cause headaches, migraines and insomnia. Getting enough sunlight and good quality, early sleep are necessary for maintaining normal mind and body cycles. In spiritual traditions, one of the basic laws of nature that enhances the activation of the seventh chakra is to awaken early in the morning and sleep early at night. Noni juice activates the pineal gland and helps produce more melatonin. (See more on Noni in Chapter 4 - Rejuvenation.)

The crown chakra is known as the spiritual centre and has to do with the expansion of consciousness. When the crown chakra opens fully, which is very rare, then a person becomes enlightened, they are literally filled with light and radiance. It is from the crown chakra that our spiritual and higher aspirations come, the desire to do spiritual work, to fulfil one's life purpose and to live one's personal truth.

The crown centre is very sensitive and affected by magnetic fields or bad vibrations. Any form of agitation, stress or emotional discord will prevent this centre from opening or even damage it. To aid in the development of this centre, we need to provide the right sort of nourishment through spiritual practises, spending time in nature in order to receive prana, eating sattvic, pure and wholesome foods and cultivating a higher awareness. A fully developed, enlightened person would wish to maintain the highest level of vibration and would therefore have no desire to eat or drink or engage in a lifestyle that is not sattvic and pure.

Disorders of the seventh chakra include nervous system disorders, paralysis, autism and debilitating diseases. It must be remembered that each chakra is affected and influenced by the other chakras and no chakra works in isolation. The crown chakra normally opens after all the other chakras have opened and this requires a great deal of inner, conscious work as well as attention to lifestyle and habits. The seventh chakra is influenced by the level of development of harmony and inner peace, which are attained through meditation, deep self-reflection and a refined state of beingness. When the seventh chakra opens completely, outer events no longer have an affect on one's inner state, which has already become established in samadhi, joy and bliss. The root chakra grounds this experience into every day life.

To move to higher levels of consciousness, it is necessary to give up all harmful substances that produce a detrimental affect on the body and the mind and to avoid people and places with low vibrations that can drag you down to their level if you are not strong enough. Spending time in nature is nurturing, looking at the sky and stars, or sitting on the top of mountains can give you the experience of vastness, expansiveness and boundlessness that can also be developed inside. Fasting is said to be helpful in opening the seventh chakra but longer fasts should not be attempted until the body and mind have already been well purified.

The colours violet, white and gold are associated with the crown chakra.

The Yoga asana for the crown chakra is the headstand. Most people, especially westerners are not ready for the headstand unless they have been practising Yoga for many years, but they can practise the introduction to the headstand, which is safe unless they have mental disorders or high blood pressure. Sitting in full or half lotus position in meditation is the position to receive higher vibrations and to open one's consciousness.

10 - THE WOUNDED WOMAN

Every woman wants to blossom and to live her full potential, what holds her back are the shadows and unfinished business from the past. Holding onto suppressed and unresolved issues takes a lot of energy; it keeps us stuck and prevents us from moving forward. When we release these blockages and the stagnant energy that is held within them, a newfound freedom gushes forth. Beneath the self imposed limitations lies a wealth of untapped potential and creativity that longs to emerge.

Most women have within them a wounded woman who has at some time felt pain or suffered in some way. It is rare to go through life without experiencing a rejection, a loss, disillusionment or a disappointment; these are all a part of life. It is not so much what happens but the way we handle these experiences that makes the difference. We can stay conscious, integrate our experiences and release them or go into denial and hold onto them. If you hold onto hurt from the past and let it build up, layer upon layer, it creates anger and resentment, which festers and generates an inner state of sourness that literally poisons the body. By continuously identifying with pain and the part of us that feels wounded; we disempower ourselves and fall into the role of the victim.

Healing the wounds of the heart is the greatest work we can do and no one else can do it for us. All feelings of sadness, loneliness or feeling unloved need to be identified, transformed and transmuted. In the Course in Miracles, it says that we are never upset for the reason we think. If you look deeper, you will discover core issues that you need to work with, negative patterns and belief systems about yourself that keep you stuck. Many of these can be traced back to childhood and the beliefs which your parents or those around you had, which may have been right for them at that time but did not necessarily synthesize with the essence of who you really are. Feelings of not being understood, appreciated or loved in the way that you needed may have led to low self-esteem or not feeling good enough.

There are also karmic threads, which come from other lifetimes, which need to be cleared. If you find that you keep repeating certain patterns, there is most likely a karmic situation involved. These threads from the past can be released. By paying attention to your emotional state and recognizing and coming to grips with any emotional discord, you can identify your patterns and transform them. The work of deep self-transformation begins with being more watchful of your thoughts and feelings in order to transform negative discord, and gradually moving to a higher vibrational level and more enlightened way of being. Negative emotions create a chemical reaction in the body, which can alter brain chemistry, disturb the nervous system and upset the hormonal flow. Bad posture, back pain, round shoulders, shallow breathing and contracted muscles are all symptoms of emotional holding. The healing process can be likened to peeling back the layers of an onion. We peel back layer upon layer of emotional holding, tension and stress, until we reach the true core and set ourselves free.

Every thought, feeling and experience is registered in the body, if we keep choosing to suppress or ignore our feelings, at some point they will surface in an unexpected way or create disease in the body. The past can block our present and interfere with our future. Unresolved issues from past relationships will bring up similar issues in your present relationships and cloud your vision of life. Through healing the past, you can reclaim your true sense of self and open to your full potential.

Psychologists spend years trying to help people sort out their past and release their pain and traumas. A good therapist can help you see where you are stuck and help you open doors that you may have been afraid to look behind or to gain a clearer perspective on different issues in your life. This can help you move beyond your fears and recognize old patterns of behaviour that no longer serve you. In my own training as a Psychosynthesis therapist, which is a transpersonal psychotherapy, we were trained to look deeply into ourselves so as to come to know our many different aspects. In doing so, we encountered the dark and the light, the dark being our shadow and the light, the transpersonal, the higher aspects of ourselves. We learnt how to bring in the light and shine it like a torch in order to transform the darker parts of ourselves.

The shadow is the part of us, which is either unconscious or what might be referred to as the undesirable parts of ourselves that we would rather not see or acknowledge. It contains an accumulation of everything we have ignored or suppressed. We have to be careful of not indulging in the past, for we can go on digging and digging into the unconscious forever, pulling out mountains of stuff without ever feeling any better. Certainly it can be helpful to share your pain and discomfort in order to get a clearer perspective but you also have to empower yourself to move beyond the limitations of the past. By identifying your major core issues and patterns, the real tranformative work can begin.

In transpersonal psychotherapies, the focus includes also embracing the spiritual domain as an important part in the search for self-realization and self-actualisation. When you work within the transpersonal realm, you can gain access to the higher self and to implement the wisdom that is given on a daily basis. This is the process of growing into your divine presence and the fullness and richness of who you really are, a radiant woman in your own right.

Through acknowledging that there is a source from whence all divine inspiration flows, you can allow it to begin working in its wonderful and mysterious ways that can bring miracles into your life. This source is totally indefinable and beyond the comprehension of our limited, human mind. It is the universal consciousness, expansive and immeasurable, ready to guide and support and to help you transform, if you would become more aware, embrace and align with it.

So much energy gets tied up in the past; wanting to turn the clock back or wishing things had turned out differently. This attachment to the past, conscious or not, blocks us from moving forwards. You have to undo the shackles of the past and free yourself. Unfulfilled dreams and disappointments in life can create a sense of loss or the feeling of having missed out. When you access this place of deep longing and go into the void, you will discover that beyond the emptiness, there is also a richness and a fullness waiting to come forward.

Deep within every human being lies the desire to be happy, to love and be loved. If you hold the love back, you feel unfulfilled or suppressed. In opening the heart and releasing and forgiving what has gone before, you not only allow yourself the opportunity to love again but you will also attract to you those who will support, love and appreciate you.

When you go through a difficult or upsetting experience, you basically have two choices of action. You can either close down and cut off because it is too painful, this means remaining in a state of pain and sadness, or you can choose to stay open, feel what is there, grieve if necessary for a period of time and then when you are ready, release, heal and transform. In the second way, you are aware of the past, you have not suppressed it, but dealt with it consciously. This then allows you to open again to the sweetness of life, to dare to love again and to regain wholeness.

The key to spiritual healing is unconditional love. Learning to love and forgive yourself and others for anything that has occurred in the past is of the utmost importance. This can be better understood once you have released any expectations of others that you may have held, if you expected them to behave in a certain way and they could not live up to your expectations, this may have left you feeling disappointed or rejected. You have to understand that they acted from their level of awareness and consciousness at the time and could not necessarily fulfil your needs.

Without forgiveness there can be no true release and the heart will remain closed. To forgive is to go beyond and to have compassion both for yourself and for others. Unfinished business from the past creates fragmentation. It is always there in the background, tugging at your emotions and taking your energy. It is excess baggage. By letting go of judgement and accepting that what is done is done, over and past, you free yourself to live totally in the present and to open to new experiences, which are no longer restrained by the past and unfinished business. By living in the present and accepting what is, you can come from a place of fullness rather than lack.

Everyone needs attention, appreciation and love but we cannot demand it from others, we have to accept people as they are with their inadequacies and limitations, just as we have our own. If you feel neglected or lacking emotional nourishment, then you must find ways to nourish yourself and not expect others to give it to you. By constantly dwelling on the past and what happened or comparing things to the past, you keep yourself stuck by moving round and round the same circle. Constant identification with pain brings self-pity and the endless cycle of victim consciousness, which locks you into an uncomfortable pattern.

Every family has experienced a tragedy of some sort or knows someone who has, but no matter how hard it is, life must go on. Life is too short and we never know what is around the corner or when it will come to an end. Death is always lurking somewhere in the background and for that very reason; you have to live a full life, now, not sometime in the future. Every day can be a new beginning, a release, a birth and a rebirth.

Beneath the wounded woman, there often lies a desperate child that is crying out for attention, comfort, love and healing. A child that felt misunderstood or unloved or that was abused or treated unfairly. By exploring the world of the inner child, you can soothe her wounds and set the wounded woman free. Maybe the grown woman needs more fun in her life, to play, to dance, to write or to sing or to do something, which would nourish her inner child. If the child felt a lack of love when growing up, she may still be looking for the ideal mother or father figure to replace the parents that did not fulfil her needs.

The adult-child may go in and out of relationships looking for a substitute mother or father. Partners sometimes fall into this trap, expecting to be parented by their partner and then if the partner does not accommodate them or behave in the way that is desired, patterns of insecurity or desperation may surface making them want to look for a new partner who will better fulfil their needs. By acknowledging the needs of your inner child and by nourishing and consoling her, you may set the wounded woman free. At some point, the child has to grow up; it can't keep looking for mummy or daddy to fix things for her. We often see adults having childish tantrums and ranting and raving when they don't get their way, then we know that inside is an unsatisfied or unhappy child.

Victim consciousness goes deep, if you hear yourself constantly justifying, moaning, whining, complaining, blaming, being critical, judgemental or resentful, then you know you are in the victim mode and this needs attention and you may need professional help to pull you out of these patterns. Everything in our past has influenced us, our upbringing, the attitudes of our parents, the society we live in, our education and the people we spend most of our time with. All these factors have helped create the patterns, attitudes and limitations that you now have. Some of those attitudes may no longer suit or serve you, you may find you have outgrown them and wish to choose new ways of evolving now, ways that are more positive, uplifting and conscious and that support you in completely leaving the victim behind.

If there is dissatisfaction, an inability to express or communicate, sadness, resentment or grief, then these things need to be addressed and resolved. Addictions, cravings, alcohol, smoking, drugs, overeating, being a workaholic or the inability to be alone, are all ways of pushing down what we don't want to see or feel. These suppressed feelings and disappointments in life lie at the root of many cancers and diseases. Drug abuse, alcoholism and serious eating disorders are a cry for help and they mask deep unresolved pain.

The roots of discontent are many; it is never just one thing that makes us unhappy. It is layers and layers of stress, rejection and unsatisfied desires that accumulate over the years. When these feelings are not discharged on a regular basis, we may suddenly find ourselves overwhelmed or depressed or exhausted and not really know why. Counselling and rebirthing are valuable tools to help release the past.

The wounded woman is always crying for attention and she wants to be loved and supported but it takes courage to reach out. If she feels neglected or misunderstood or craves love and nourishment, she may be reactive, unreasonable or moody and create dramas to get attention. She longs to express herself freely but is restricted by her own limitations, which confine her and then because she is so often unconscious of these patterns that are working within her, she blames others for her life circumstances and cannot realize that there is a way to break free and start again. This begins with self-awareness and taking responsibility for oneself. As you open to a new level of awareness, you become more accountable for your actions.

By bringing your attention to the present moment and what is happening right now and getting a sense of what needs to shift and change, you start to free your energy and discover what it means to feel free. This is reclaiming your power and as you do so, you will start to feel more alive and vital. As an observer of yourself, you have to be vigilant in maintaining your alertness, so as to catch yourself each time you slip back into old habits and patterns or victim consciousness, which are not in alignment with your new vision of how you want to be or how you want to lead your life.

By identifying your tendencies, you can create an action plan that works for you and build a support system that supports and enhances it. This support system may consist of family and friends and also professionals or teachers who may be able to guide or help you as you continue your exploration of previously unknown possibilities including becoming a spiritual woman and treading the spiritual path.

Before the radiant woman can come forth truly inspired with vision, clarity and wisdom, all emotional discord must be released or transformed. Similarly, no rejuvenation can take place until all stress, tension and discord have been dissolved. By developing a new passion for life and deciding to live fully and abundantly now, the wounded woman can be released and be like just a whisper from the past. Determination can help you break through all limiting patterns that have held you back and by holding a clear focus on what you want, you can achieve it. Assistance is always there from the angelic realms, help is always given when there is faith and trust and often comes in unexpected ways as anyone on the spiritual path can verify.

Through healing all emotional scarring and wounds of the past, the radiant woman can emerge and regain her wholeness. This era is an important time of transition, women everywhere are waking up and empowering themselves. Spiritual empowerment has nothing to do with ego, it is the natural, pure life force that comes from the depths of one's being, it is the shakti energy, the divine, feminine wisdom that is insightful, all embracing, loving and compassionate.

Healing is an ongoing process of the development of awareness. It is a process not a quick fix, which encompasses deep understanding that is combined with wisdom and embraces the expansion of consciousness. Through nurturing ourselves and allowing ourselves to be nurtured, especially by the universal source, we can uplift our vibrational level, move into higher states of consciousness and consequently change our lives. The more you turn towards the spiritual, the more you will draw to you exactly what you need to help you grow and mature spiritually. The power of the divine will give you the healing and sustenance that you need and help you find your way. Then amazingly, you will find yourself in the right place at the right time and the right people and the right circumstances will come into your life exactly when you need them.

11 - REBIRTHING - PRANIC BREATHING

Rebirthing is a powerful healing process, which works on the mental, emotional, physical and spiritual levels. It is a therapy that helps clear emotional and physical blocks from the body and releases layers and layers of tension, stress and tightly held patterns of energy from the body. It is a tool for the expansion of consciousness, freeing you from the limitations of the past. Rebirthing is also known as pranic breathing and is based upon a specific breathing technique of conscious, connected breathing.

When you first start the rebirthing process, you need to work with a rebirther, who is your personal breathing coach and support system, but later when you are comfortable and more proficient with the process, you can rebirth yourself. Your rebirther keeps you focused, alert and awake and helps you to work through anything that might come up in the session. As you move through blocks, there can be the tendency to stop or fall asleep, but your rebirther keeps you breathing and encourages you to keep going.

During a rebirthing session, one breathes for approximately one hour but some deep sessions may take longer. In the first ten sessions usually a lot of suppressed material comes to the surface to be released. Some people experience this visually and see pictures or images, whereas others just experience it as energy moving in the body or feel that they are in very deep state of relaxation, everyone's experience is different. As this is a process, it is advised if possible to have regular sessions for a period of time, this could be weekly or fortnightly. I usually recommend to my clients once they feel they have completed the initial clearing, which could be anything between ten to twenty sessions, then to come for a session at least once a month even if they are rebirthing themselves. This helps them continue to access unconscious material and to share their insights and work with core issues and specific themes of interest. It is also easier to move into higher states of consciousness when someone else keeps you focused and encourages you to move beyond your limitations.

My own personal interest and exploration of the spiritual path led me into many areas of self-development, energywork and healing. I started with Psychosynthesis and Yoga and meditation and then trained in Ayurveda, bodywork and different schools of healing. This helped me to see the important connection between holding emotional distress and the effect on the physical body. I realized that although counselling, diet and good lifestyle were all very important, we also need to work with the body in order to release traumas and emotional pain. When we work with the body as well and get the energy moving, the results are far more impressive. As emotional distress, strain and tension are released from the body, then many physical ailments clear up by themselves.

In rebirthing, there are two important factors, one is the emotional release and the other is the oxygenation of the body through the specific breathing technique of conscious, connected breathing combined with deep relaxation, which allows integration. Together they create a metamorphosis. This is in alignment with the teachings of esoteric healing, which believes that beneath all physical pain lies emotional discord and dissatisfaction. For a long time, my work seemed to be divided into two categories, the physical and the emotional. Rebirthing provided the missing link.

When you start practising pranic breathing, an ongoing circuit of energy is created, this promotes a cathartic effect, which dissolves the patterns of stress, which are held in the body from the past, including limitations, grief and fear. Suppressed emotions are activated and brought to the surface to be released. Rebirthing works both with the conscious and the unconscious and many things will be dissolved without even knowing what they are. Over a period of time, the breath is able to bring about changes on a cellular level and release memories, which are deeply imbedded in the cellular memory. The purpose of rebirthing is to free the breath so as to free the person, this moves the energy in the body and dissolves physical, emotional and energy blocks. As the energy moves, it purifies, nourishes and regenerates.

In teaching Yoga, I began to observe that most people don't breath properly, their breathing is too shallow and they tend to breath only in the chest area rather than in the abdomen. As babies we naturally breathed from the belly and the chest was relaxed. If you watch any baby or young child when they are sleeping, you will see that they breathe from the abdomen. As we get older and feel the pressures of life, stress constricts us and this affects our breathing patterns. This is unnatural and creates tension in the chest, shoulders and neck and can create headaches and migraines and many other problems. As we free the breath and release the tension from these areas, all the systems of the body are oxygenated and this improves circulation, clears out toxins and purifies the blood. Rebirthing helps accelerate this process.

Shallow breathing prevents the brain from receiving enough oxygen and this may result in fatigue, sluggishness, lack of focus and depression. The breath is the most powerful force of life, without it we cannot exist; it is the vital life force, which sustains the body. When the last breath has stopped, then life, as we know it comes to an end. Oxygen is the most vital nutrient for the body. We can do without food and water for a period of time but we cannot live without oxygen, we would die in a few minutes. Through the process of breathing, oxygen is carried to every part of the body. Rebirthing helps oxygenate the whole body and is therefore an important part of any rejuvenation programme.

Restricted breathing has to do with emotional holding and resistance, suppressing the feelings, not wanting to face something, not wanting to let go or holding tight because of fear. Your breathing reflects what's going on in you and how alive you are. When you get stressed or angry, this creates pressure and restricts your breathing and creates damage not only to the brain and the lungs but also to the whole body. Most people use only one fifth of their lung capacity. By learning to be more relaxed and improving your lung capacity, you can greatly improve your health and increase your energy level. Quick walking on a daily basis is an excellent way to expand lung capacity whereas jogging is too strenuous for many people and can create a strain on the heart. We have all seen people who jog and look exhausted and as if they are about to collapse. Over exertion, going beyond our comfortable capacity is not helpful and should be avoided. Common sense tells us that it is better to build up slowly and give the body time to adjust and gradually and slowly expand our comfort zone.

Lack of sufficient oxygen can cause major problems to the brain and the heart. The brain requires more oxygen than any other part of the body. Oxygen increases lymphatic movement and has a cleansing effect on the cells. When the cells do not receive enough oxygen, abnormalities can occur. Deprivation of oxygen is thought to play a major part in the formation of malignant and cancerous cells. Pranic breathing increases the oxygen levels in the blood and improves the quality of the blood by releasing toxins, bacteria and viruses. Lack of oxygen relates to a lack of energy.

There is nothing more destructive to the body especially to the brain than smoking. Smoking deprives the cells of oxygen and accelerates the ageing process. Smoking pollutes the body with harmful chemicals and causes degeneration and premature ageing. When there is a lack of sufficient oxygen to the brain, a stroke can occur, when the heart is deprived of oxygen, a heart attack can occur. If you look at the skin of a long-term smoker, you will see that it is dull, it does not shine or glow and it may also have a yellowish tinge because of the toxic effect on the liver.

The breathe of life is sacred, it is God given. In rebirthing, the breath is used as a release mechanism for healing to occur through the release of deep tension, anxiety and fear. Through full oxygenation of the body, healing can take place even at the level of the DNA and genetic imbalances can be influenced. Through mastering the breath, we can master ourselves.

199

As you release whatever has been suppressed or blocking, you can move into a state of bliss consciousness, this is the ultimate aim of rebirthing and a lot has been written about this state. Bliss is an inner state of ecstasy, an ongoing state of joy, which is not influenced or affected by outer circumstances. In the beginning, you may start to experience fleeting moments of bliss and then as you get clearer, these experiences increase. The same state can be accessed through meditation. You cannot feel bliss or pure joy if you blocked by past, unintegrated experiences. Joy and bliss are the natural birthright of everyone.

Rebirthing offers a simple way to unmask, free and release oneself from the burdens of the past and to learn how to continue doing this on a daily basis, so as not to build up layers of stress and tension again. It is also a way to reveal our true nature. At the core of our being, beneath all the conditioning and false beliefs and suppressed material, we can discover a state of purity, innocence and a powerful reservoir of energy. Yogis have long known the amazing tranformative power of working with the breath and they practise specific pranayamas (breathing techniques) to fully oxygenate the body in order to rejuvenate. They consider prana, which is taken in with the breath to be the spiritual sustenance of the universe. Some Yogis are breatharians, they take no food and live and exist only on the breath.

During a rebirthing session, you move into a state of deep relaxation and become more aware of the breath and the body. By observing what is happening in the body and quickening the breath, your awareness becomes sharper and you feel more acutely the places where you hold tension and tightness in the body. You begin to feel the fluctuations of energy as it releases and moves through the body. Sometimes this makes the body twitch or jerk or jump. Sometimes strong pulsating waves of energy move quickly through the body. Many memories may be activated and past situations and people may come into your mind as a way of integrating the experience. With on-going sessions, the tension and old energy patterns from the past begin to unwind, then as you look back, you realize how much you were holding and suppressing. After each session time is given for integration. Old structures have been dismantled and the space for something new has been created. Curling up on one side in the fetal position for a few minutes whilst integrating feels comfortable and soothing.

Clients always tell me how much better they feel after a few sessions. In some people the changes come slowly; in others the changes are visible almost straight away. Over the weeks and months with constant unwinding and releasing, a new feeling of inner freedom and relief is felt. When you hold yourself back, you restrict the expression of your full potential and the joy and bliss that wants to flow through. To free yourself, you first have to free the breath. Pay attention to your breathing and notice how it is restricted or how it changes whenever you get upset.

Prana, the healing energy has the ability to purify, regenerate and heal. As the energy flows more freely through the body, it acts as a detoxifier as it clears and cleans debris from the body. With more life force moving through the body, the chakras may then become activated and this will increase the feeling of aliveness. By relaxing deeply into the process and focusing on the breath, you can let go of all struggle, pain and fear and even phobias can be overcome. Rebirthing is deep, tranformative, emotional release work; it clears the way to connect to deeper levels of the self. Gradually the body armour, which has been set up as a protection over the years is dissolved. This armour keeps you stuck in a tight, restrictive pattern and limited mode of functioning. These defence mechanisms limit your potential and prevent the natural flow of expression.

When rebirthing first became popular about twenty years ago, much of the focus was on the birth trauma. Although this is an important aspect of the work, many therapists, myself included, no longer focus specifically on this area. If and when the birth trauma comes up in a session, then it will be integrated. Because of this shift and the changes that have occurred in this field of work, some therapists now refer to their work as Breath Therapy, Pranic breathing or Conscious Connected breathing. Like all therapies, Rebirthing has evolved considerably in the last ten years. What is the most important is finding the right therapist to work with, someone whom you trust and feel comfortable with, always go by your intuition.

For me rebirthing has become an important part of my practise and combines well with meditation and Yoga. I see rebirthing as a gentle release and explorative process to be used on a daily basis to release any accumulated strain or stress from the day. When you clear at the end of the day, you feel fresher and more vibrant the next day. It also helps improve the quality of your sleep. Meditation followed by fifteen minutes (or longer) of rebirthing every day can be a powerful combination and at least one longer session per week. (This is after you have done a course of major clearing sessions with a rebirther). Rebirthing can lead you into higher states of consciousness and into more expansive and unlimited parts of yourself.

The reason the birth trauma was considered such an important factor in rebirthing is because it is believed that birth is a traumatic experience for everyone. Leaving the comfort and safety of the womb, being pushed down the birth canal and then out into the world can be an uncomfortable and traumatic experience for both the child and the mother and especially if the child is taken away from the mother too soon. It is now known how important it is not to cut the umbilical cord too soon so the child has time to adjust to its new surroundings. When the cord is cut too soon, or the child is taken away from the mother at birth this may create feelings of being unloved, isolation or fear. This is why research now shows that premature babies in an incubator should be touched and stroked as much as possible by the parents.

Although there is a lot more awareness today around natural childbirth, very few babies are now born at home in a nurturing environment and clinical environments with bright lights and loud noises are hostile to the child. Although medicine has progressed tremendously in this field and very few women die in childbirth in comparison to the past, there is now a growing concern about the amount of drugs including epidurals, which are given to women routinely, which may affect the baby. There are times when these procedures may be necessary and life saving but often they are used as clinical procedures to quicken the process for the convenience of the doctor instead of letting nature take its natural course We must remember that childbirth and breastfeeding are natural God given processes and therefore should be interfered with as little as possible. Our first impressions and associations from birth are carried with us throughout the whole of our lives and this is why the birth trauma needs to be released. The birth trauma may have created fear, which gets locked in the memory and the cells. When people release their birth trauma, they can totally release themselves.

There is a connection between the quality of your breath and the quality of your life. Our concept of life, our thoughts and ideas about ourselves began whilst we were still in the womb. A lot has been written about the impressions and influences upon the unborn child. Everything has a profound effect on the child including the relationship between the parents, whether the pregnancy was wanted and the mother's attitude to the child during pregnancy. Children that are consciously conceived, carried in a loving way and have a natural birth are more likely to be happier and healthier and successful in life.

The release of the birth trauma is known as the breath release. The breath release is a major, tranformative experience. It may take a lot of work to reach the breath release or it may happen suddenly and spontaneously. Unconsciously we all seek to return to the comfort and safety of the womb and to be nourished by the universe again. This is why we want to be nurtured by others when we are feeling low. Being tucked up in a warm bed makes us feel safe and comfortable especially when we are not feeling well, it reminds us of the womb experience. That is why people who are severely depressed want to stay in bed all day or don't want to get up in the morning.

Warm water, baths, whirlpools, natural warm springs and even warm showers give a similar feeling of comfort. For this reason, rebirthing is also done in warm water tubs. Warm water calms us when we are stressed and helps release the tension out of the body. Lying in the bath, listening to soothing music and doing connected, conscious breathing can be very soothing but be careful not to drift off to sleep or to go into a deep rebirthing experience if you are alone. It is advisable to have someone with you if you are rebirthing in water.

Rebirthing is a helpful tool in any rejuvenation programme because it oxygenates and enlivens the whole body including all the organs and the brain. When we take in enough prana and oxygen, which is the food of the universe, then the nervous system and every cell is nourished, the blood is purified and many physical problems including addictions, anorexia, arthritis, asthma, menstrual disorders and migraines can be transformed. Suppression and emotional holding cause stagnation and are the root cause of many diseases.

Working with the power of the mind and our thoughts is another aspect of rebirthing. Using affirmations helps transform limited thought patterns and negative beliefs and uncovers weaknesses and destructive tendencies. All limiting thought patterns come from the past. By uncovering core beliefs and reprogramming your thoughts, you can recreate, change and redirect your life. We have been conditioned to think like our parents and the way society wants us to think and when this doesn't feel right we want to rebel and break free from these limiting constraints. The world is a mirror of our thoughts; we create what we think about. Once you understand the power and the consequences of your thoughts, this opens you to infinite possibilities. You have within you the ability to become a conscious creator; the question is what do you want to create?

In my own practise I combine rebirthing with healing and find this a very powerful and effective way to work and I would like to see more healers doing the same and plan to start trainings in this area of work. Through rebirthing you can move from fear into love, from lack into fullness, from pain to joy and from limitations to the unlimited. Through realizing and mastering the power of the breath, you can do the same with your life and experience bliss consciousness.

12 - SELF HEALING – NURTURING THE SELF

Self-healing comes from deep self-nurturing, it means giving yourself the love, attention and care that you need. It starts with taking full responsibility for your health and your life and not blaming others or circumstances for the events that have taken place. From now on, you can decide to make choices that support, nourish and enrich you in every way. This is not selfish, it is about improving the quality of your life and becoming the person you long to be through living your full potential. This naturally includes taking care of your health and well-being. When you do this, you will feel happier and more fulfilled and want to support and nourish those around you in the same way. This means speaking and living your truth and transforming any negative aspects of yourself.

The secret is to transform through love, loving yourself for who you are at this point in time, with all your faults, exactly as you are right now. You need to forgive yourself for the mistakes you made in the past, let them go, try not to repeat them and move on. Loving yourself means doing things that make you happy. We cannot heal if we live a life of untruths or pretence. If you are in a relationship that is not working, your truth may be that it is time to move on. If you are in a job that you do not like or are only there for the money, it may be time to change it.

Usually when we want to make major life changes, a lot of fear comes up and that fear can keep us stuck in uncomfortable and unfulfilling circumstances for the rest of our lives. As you challenge yourself to move through the fear and discomfort and maybe take some risks, you will feel more alive. Living your truth and expressing it, sets you free and is an important part of any healing process. When you stay locked in a pattern of fear, nothing moves, the energy remains stagnant. This is where rebirthing is such a valuable tool, once you have done a series of rebirthing sessions, you can then regularly rebirth yourself and keep moving through patterns of fear as they come up and shift the energy that is associated with those fears. Once you have sorted one issue and then the next, you will see that it is not so difficult after all and you can deal with core issues and shift deep rooted patterns that may have been holding you back for years.

Self-realization and self-healing go hand in hand. It is a process of spiritual alchemy, of transforming ourselves from one state to another. We can move from limitations to unlimitedness, from low self esteem to empowerment, from pain to love and from unhappiness to bliss. There are no limitations to what you can achieve; it just depends on how far you want to go. The potential is always there in an unmanifest form waiting to be expressed.

Women often feel guilty when they do something for themselves, they are so used to giving to others, to their husbands, children, families and friends that they often neglect themselves. Tiredness, stress and on-going tension are all evidence of self-neglect. If you lead a busy and active life, then you have to get things in perspective and all the more reason, to take time for yourself. Women are the nurturers but they have to remember to nurture themselves. Depending on what you can afford, give yourself a regular gift of a weekly or monthly treatment, healing, reflexology, massage, rebirthing or something that will nourish you. If money is a restriction at this time, then find ways to do an exchange. Try different options until you find what suits you, it will make you feel special and it is a way of appreciating yourself. You deserve it, when you do something special for yourself, it makes you feel good and that feeling flows through into every area of your life and those close to you will benefit too.

Although it is good to become self sufficient and to be able to stand firmly on your own two feet, you also need friends and different people who will support you and be there for you when you need it. Part of my spiritual service and support work, is co-ordinating the Global Spiritual Network on the Internet. For many years I managed the Women's Spiritual Network and recently it evolved into the GSN. Every day I send out free postings to thousands of people all over the world on subjects relating to spirituality, health and healing. The purpose of this is to share information, inspire and uplift and transform consciousness. In return, I connect with many interesting people in different countries and get invited to give seminars and people send me interesting information, which they want to share. It is a way of creating a global spiritual family and circulating good energy and goodwill. If you wish to join the GSN and receive the daily postings contact me at surya@spidernet.com.cy.

Creating a deep connection with different people is nourishing and helps us to expand our horizons and to evolve. Good friends are there to help each other and that is how friendships develop. It may be time to let go of superficial friendships or people you no longer have so much in common with, this happens as you grow and move on. Some friends stay for a lifetime, others move in and out of our lives and we should not be afraid to let them go when the time is right. When you give up on shoulds and obligations (that does not mean not being there for those who need your help and support) then you have more free time to do the things you really like and consciously choose who you want to spend time with.

Your support network might include professional people too, like a counsellor, healer or rebirther. You will find that at different times you are drawn to different people and when you listen to your deeper needs, your inner presence will draw to you what is needed. Sometimes you have to let go of things before something new can come into your life. Letting go is never easy but it is very freeing and opens you to new possibilities in your life. Your time is precious, so don't waste it by spending time with people you don't really want to be with, this creates resentment, which can turn to frustration and anger.

The first half of this book is about healing through taking care of your physical needs; the second half is about healing on an energy level and addressing your emotional needs. Detoxification needs to take place not only physically and emotionally but also mentally. Mental detoxification means releasing old programmes and thought patterns that no longer serve you and replacing them with new, positive, productive ways of thinking and being, this is called repatterning or reprogramming. If you go on thinking in the same way, you will get the same results and not much will change. The same thoughts will create the same situations; therefore you need to work on a mental level to bring about the desired changes. When you engage in a mental detox programme, you have to be willing to be totally honest with yourself in order to identify the patterns that need to change. You can release negative and limiting thought patterns and replace them with more positive, uplifting and creative thoughts. This can turn your whole life around.

The following are recommended for a mental detox programme:

- No more whining, complaining, blaming others, going into victim consciousness or poor me. Instead look for solutions, there is always a way even if you cannot see it yet.
- No struggle, no strain, no pain. Learning to go with the flow, to accept what is happening in the moment and to hold the faith that you can create something better for the future. Don't struggle with anything, allow and be with it until you get new insights. Don't let negative thoughts come in and sabotage.
- No doubt, fear or despair. Replacing these with trust in a higher power, the unseen spiritual force which comes to our aid and guides us when we open to it.
- No attachment. It is our attachment to people, things and certain outcomes that cause us pain or block our progress. When we let go, new people come to our lives and unexpected things happen. Expect the unexpected.
- No lack. Moving out of the pattern of lack into abundance, clearing old patterns of lack from your life.
- No shoulds. Instead of living a life of shoulds, make choices, choose to do things willingly and always do your best.
- No energy drains. Not allowing yourself to overwork or to push yourself beyond your physical or emotional capabilities. Remember your health comes first. Not allowing others to

make unfair demands upon you or to drain your energy. Instead nourish yourself and ask for support when you need it.

- No self-abuse. Not taking substances into your body, which you know are harmful or not good for you. Not doing things, which are not in your best interest or spending time with people who are negative or bring you down. Not putting yourself down or being angry for things that have happened in the past or don't work out the way you want, instead work on forgiving, loving and appreciating yourself.

- No dramas. Don't go into childish dramas, moodiness or tantrums in order to get what you want and don't get pulled into other peoples' dramas either. All dramas are manipulation and a way of trying to get control. Instead practise open, honest, clear communication.

- No attacking, criticizing, blaming or judgement. Everyone has their stuff, let them get on with it and concentrate on your own growth work and what you can do.

- Don't compare, we are all unique individuals. Discover your own talents and gifts and put them to work.

Repatterning and reprogramming

Repatterning and reprogramming are a constant on going process. As you work on one area and sort it out, then you will find other things that need attention too, this is how the process of transformation occurs, step-by-step, moment-by-moment. Don't get discouraged if it feels like there is so much work to be done, there is, for all of us but the results are wonderful and fulfilling. Self-work not only transforms your life but it can also expand further out and create a better world to live in. Each of us has a part to play in a greater plan, we do what we can and then it extends out, often touching others in unknown or unexpected ways. We never know where our circle of influence, positive energy, inspiration or joy might reach.

Positive reprogramming includes the following:

- Nourish yourself in every possible way and take full responsibility for yourself and your life and what you create.
- Learn to live effortlessly, to go with the flow, not to fight against it, allowing and accepting but constantly being alert to new opportunities and possibilities.
- Expect the unexpected, always be ready, you never know what is just round the corner or what this day may bring.
- Develop the qualities of joy, love, bliss and grace.
- Love and appreciate others and they will love and appreciate you.
- Be open to fresh ideas and new ways of doing things, allow your creativity to flow and live your full potential.
- Open to abundance consciousness.
- Be positive, have an enthusiasm for life and trust the process.
- Nurture your friendships and develop a good support system.
- Communicate honestly and live your truth.
- Live with vision, create the life you desire and don't be influenced by those who have limited vision. Spend time with those who nourish, encourage and support you. Continually seek out people with more knowledge or a higher consciousness so that you can learn from them.
- Develop a spiritual practise and maintain it. The divine connection offers the greatest nourishment and is there for you at all times, no matter where you are.

In the morning, take a few minutes to plan your day, not just the things you have to do but how you want to be. This helps you cultivate the qualities that you need to develop in yourself, to stay centered, be more open and focused, compassionate, patient etc. The clearer you are about your intention, the more you can bring it into being. If nothing goes according to plan or everything gets turned upside down, be open and spontaneous, take it as a creative challenge but do not allow it to upset or disturb you. As you watch yourself and your behaviour, you can observe how you respond and whether you are able to remain centered and keep your cool or whether you react and become upset. The more you watch and monitor your responses and reactions, the clearer your patterns will become and then you can choose to act differently.

In the evening, take a few minutes to review your day and see how it went, play it back in your mind like a film. See what stands out. What went well that you can be pleased with or was there anything you would like to have done differently. What can you learn from today's experiences?

Affirmations are very helpful in changing mental patterns and getting to the root of what lies underneath. Keep working on a chosen affirmation until you feel that the new pattern is firmly established in your life. For example if you are working on creating radiant health, you might affirm, "I am radiant and healthy". As you do this, you will start to become more aware of your habits that interfere with your being radiant and healthy. Then you might look deeper as to why you have these habits, what are the emotions that lie behind them that make you behave in a certain way and what do you need to do to heal them.

If you are working on being more positive or joyful, for example "I am always positive and joyful", you will start to notice whenever you are not feeling positive and joyful and work with the causes. Avoid negativity; refuse to engage in gossip or negative conversations about others, by doing this you refuse to allow negativity to come into your life. You could use the affirmation "I am open and positive and draw new positive people into my life that uplift and inspire me." Then gradually you will release anything that is not in alignment with this affirmation and new people will come into your life that are more positive and inspiring.

Writing helps ground the affirmation more firmly in your consciousness. You can write the affirmation every day ten times or more until you feel it really working in your life, then you go onto the next one. Affirmations are very powerful. People who think that affirmations don't work, either have not worked with them for long enough or have not worked with the counter reactive patterns that they bring up, which prevent the pattern from working. If for example you work with, "I appreciate and love myself," everything in you that does not agree with this will rise to the surface to be cleared. If you felt unloved by your parents or your partner left you, there may still be unresolved issues such as resentment to work on.

Rebirthing and counselling can help you sort these patterns out. When you resolve patterns around lack of self-esteem and appreciate and love yourself, you will feel your worth and then draw to you people who will feel the same about you. Life is a mirror, a reflection of what is inside, you attract to you certain people and circumstances to help you work out certain things, when those patterns are completed or transformed or there is no longer anything to learn from the relationship, the person may leave your life or you may move on.

Opening the heart is the most important psychological process that facilitates healing. If we allow pain and disappointment to close us down, then we close to life and this can be likened to a slow death. Both sorrow and joy are all around us, they are a part of life just as birth and death are. When we open our hearts, we open to life and rekindle the spirit within and feel our aliveness.

Karma is the result of samskaras of the past, the seeds of discontent and wrong doings that we have done in this lifetime and past lifetimes. Discord and disharmony create karma and sow the seeds of illnesses. Unexplained illnesses or sudden deaths are most often related to karma. The release and transformation of karma comes through conscious right living and not harming others, neither through thought, word or deed. This helps balance the scales and diminish karma. Being of service to mankind and helping others in the most simple of ways creates good karma. As we work deeply on ourselves, we can ask for karma to be cleared and what we need to do to achieve this.

As we look for tools to help us in the healing process, we realize that almost anything can be therapeutic. Being in nature is very therapeutic. If you live in a city go to a park. Walking helps us integrate our experiences and to come to terms with things and let go. Go to little cafes or places where the energy feels good. Go alone as often as possible, so you can sit quietly with your thoughts, writing or just watching people and enjoying. Going to places alone teaches you to be more self-sufficient and not to always depend on being with other people.

Absorb the prana whenever you are in nature; watch the sunset, look at the sky, the moon and the stars. Follow the cycles of the moon and become aware of how the moon affects you. Find out what nurtures you the most and bring more of it into your life. Discover the sacred in every day living and enjoy it day by day, moment by moment by becoming more sensitive to what is around you and allow life to nurture you.

Music can be very healing; the importance of music in depression has been well documented and different types of music create different moods and effects. Lying in a bath scented with essential oils, candles burning and listening to soothing music can dissolve the stress from the day and bring a feeling of peace and harmony. Sound has a powerful effect on the nervous system and can help us break through patterns of fear and shift deep-seated blocks. Chanting has been used as a healing technique in many traditions over the centuries. Chanting specific sounds has a vibrational effect on the cellular level and can promote healing of the organs, tissues and cells. Each organ and chakra resonates with a specific sound. Sick organs and cells have a low, inharmonious vibration, through chanting we can lift our vibrations and bring the body back to harmony.

The two most profound healing sounds are AUM and OM. AUM is used for healing of the self and OM is a more universal sound for creating eternal peace, oneness and unity. A (pronounced AH) the first letter of AUM is associated with rebirth and new beginnings. Pregnant women in India chant AUM throughout the day to have a harmonious pregnancy and to ensure the good health of the baby. If you practise meditation, it is very good to chant AUM for five to ten minutes before meditating to cleanse the aura and to release any negative vibrations. Mantras are specific sacred sounds, which are usually given by a teacher and silently repeated in meditation.

The Tibetan chakra chant, lam, vam, ram, yam, ham, om, soham enlivens each of the chakras and the corresponding glands and organs. Lam resonates with the base chakra, vam with the second chakra, ram with the solar plexus, yam with the heart, ham with the throat, om with the third eye and soham with the crown chakra. You can bring your attention to each area as you make the related sound. Doing seven rounds of chakra chanting beginning from the base and moving upwards restores harmony between all the chakras and gets the energy moving through the whole body. Chanting every day produces profound vibrational changes and can heal many ailments in the body.

Writing is another useful tool for clearing the past. You can write down whatever you feel, expressing your deepest feelings, saying all the things you never dared say to anyone, this helps undo some of the knots inside. Then throw the paper away, you don't need to reread it or to dwell on it, just use it as an exercise for clearing and learning how to express your deepest truth.

The Metamorphic technique is a system that evolved out of reflexology and works on the principle that by stimulating certain points on the sides of the feet, the hand and the head, you can activate the whole body through the spinal connections and stimulate and balance the nervous system.

Developing a regular spiritual practice is the framework upon which all true healing is based. Without it, there cannot be any real clear introspection or depth of understanding as to where the real causes of our distress and dismay lie. Below the obvious psychological and emotional turmoil, which need to be released, there are deeper, unconscious core issues, which need to become conscious and transformed.

All the great teachers, yogis and masters have dedicated themselves to this work of the unmasking of the true self. Through aligning yourself with a higher source of power and invoking divine love, you can clear what stands in the way and connect to the radiance of the sacred within and allow the Radiant Woman to emerge. When one transcends the limitations of lower vibrations and moves into full radiance, healing can spontaneously take place of all levels. The work of self-realization and self-transformation takes dedication, patience and perseverance but its results are incomparable.

Visualization and meditation are extremely valuable tools as a part of any health and healing programme. People meditate for many different reasons, to become calm, release stress, to improve their health, to heal physical problems, to increase their mental abilities and creativity, to explore deeper within themselves, for spiritual growth, to attain higher states of consciousness and to experience wholeness and unity with the divine. Whatever the reason that you are drawn to meditation, you will receive profound insights and benefits.

I have created a series of 5 CDs, to assist your journey of health and healing. These can be listened to again and again as a way of nurturing and healing yourself. For the best results, it is recommended to listen and work with the CDs in the order given. The first is an important preparation for the other CDs.

The first CD is called **"Deep Relaxation, Moving into Stillness"**.
Learning how to deeply relax and unwind stress and tension from everyday living is essential. As you learn to relax the different parts of your body, you can move into inner stillness and feel more at peace within yourself. This CD can also be played just before sleeping to improve the quality of your sleep.

The second CD is **"Opening the Heart and Healing the Wounds of the Past."**
Through opening the heart and learning to forgive, you can heal the wounds of the past and open to new levels of yourself. Using the Violet Flame for healing, you can engage in karmic cleansing and

transform emotional discord. When you do emotional and karmic cleansing, you can remove psychological barriers that have been created and open to a higher level of vibration, the vibration of love.

The third CD is **"Healing on a Cellular Level."**
In this CD, we call upon the healing energy to cleanse, nourish and restore harmony in every cell of the body. The power of the mind should never be underestimated in its ability to heal especially when it is attuned to the highest source for healing. In this visualization, attention is drawn to the cellular level, to help reach the root cause of imbalances. Different coloured rays are used to help heal sick or weak areas of the body.

The fourth CD is **"A Chakra Meditation, for Total Balance and Harmony."**
This CD is to restore balance on all levels, between the body, mind and spirit, as well as aligning all the chakras and increasing the energy flow between them. Using guided visualization and sound you can balance and increase the vibrational rate of each chakra, as well as the glands and body parts, which are associated with each chakra.

The fifth CD is "The **Bliss Experience**."
It is recommended to work with the Bliss Experience after you have worked with the other CDs for a period of time. In this way, you will already know how to relax deeply and have cleared many limitations, which might block the bliss experience. The Bliss Experience is a combination of meditation and affirmations to move you into a state of bliss.

Space Clearing

As well as clearing yourself, it is also important to regularly clear the space that you live in. Clearing out clutter, can make a huge difference. Throw out old clothes, anything that you don't really like or need or that is broken and can't be fixed. Throw out books, old magazines, old letters and even photos. When you clutter your space with stuff from the past, you remain attached, when you clear it out, you free yourself for new things to come into your life. As clutter is removed, it makes it easier to clean the house. Cleanliness is very important. When you regularly clean your space, you freshen it up and remove any bad vibrations or negative energy that may be lurking around.

By throwing out all the old junk you have been holding onto and cleaning well, you can create sacred space. The space you live in, reflects your inner world, it is an expression of you. Create sacred space by putting lots of flowers and plants (get rid of any dying plants or dried flowers, which are considered to be bad Feng Shui). Burn essential oils and incense and add crystals to purify the area but remember to wash them regularly as they absorb negative energy. Add life to your space by making it homely, so that it is a place that you love to come home to, your sanctuary. Let it reflect you and be selective in the colours you choose. As you change, you may find you need to change things in your environment, move things around, bring in new colours or even move house or area. You can outgrow a place, just like you can outgrow a relationship.

Weekend Renewal Programme

Every now and then, it is beneficial to take some time off for a weekend renewal programme. If this is difficult because you have young children, see if you can make an arrangement with a friend and take turns to look after each other's children or ask family members to help. If this is still not possible, then at least try to find a way to have one whole, free day, which is just for you, to spend the day just for yourself. As children get older and can take more responsibility for themselves, this gets easier. Where possible, it is better to actually go away occasionally for a weekend to recharge and renew.

A weekend away could entail a self-development weekend of some sort or a meditation weekend of just being quiet, allowing and being. Weekend renewal programmes are powerful when you go alone and remove yourself completely from all contact with friends or family (just let them know what you are doing so they don't worry).

Switch your phone off during this time and don't watch TV and try not to think about work or things you have to do, this is a chance for a mental and emotional detox too. When you take time away from your usual routine, it is an opportunity for deep introspection, to see how you feel and what comes up for you. When you are alone and there is nothing to distract you, things come to the surface and stare you in the face and this gives you a clearer perspective of any changes that you need to make. Remember that your health comes first, so give yourself enough time to rest, relax and rejuvenate; this nurtures you and is an essential part of any self-healing programme.

13 - METAMORPHOSIS

The information on health and healing that has been offered in this book is the result of over twenty years of work and research. It is by no means a final, complete picture, there is always the need to explore and learn more, and it is an ongoing and exciting journey. It takes time to integrate new ideas and to absorb them into your life. You cannot change everything all at once, but little by little you can make the necessary changes and greatly improve your health and well-being and transform your life.

You can emerge, like the butterfly out of the cocoon and open like the tiny rosebud into full bloom. Radiant health is the greatest gift you can give yourself and you now have many tools to work with to help you achieve it. Eat consciously, choose sattvic and healthy food, take care of your digestion and assimilation and follow the rules of conscious eating. Rest well and sleep early so as to regenerate and heal and avoid tiring or overworking. Listen to your body and take care of your basic needs and nourish yourself well, you deserve it. Keep your stress levels to a minimum and learn to recharge yourself through relaxation, rebirthing and meditation on a daily basis. Release and transform all emotional discord so that you may discover the joy and bliss that are hidden within.

Create a support circle and invite new people into your life. At the same time become self-sufficient and strengthen your spiritual connection with the divine. As you connect more and more to your inner wisdom, your knowingness and intuition will become strong and clear so that you will naturally gravitate towards that which is sattvic, enriching and supportive of the highest ways of living and being. This will enable you to let go of everything that is not supportive of your highest good and to draw to you whatever is right for you in the moment. Know that the metamorphosis has already begun.

As you move into the fullness of your being, a new radiance will come forth that will fill you with joy and bliss. Create an ideal image of the radiant woman that you wish to become and see yourself transforming into that image.

True beauty comes from inside, it is derived from a well-nourished body, a clear mind, balanced emotions and living a harmonious life. When all discord has been cleared, you will discover a great sense of peace that is powerful and all embracing. This will enable you, to move beyond all barriers into the infinite as you find a new freedom that allows your potential to flow through and your spirit to fly. Remember that you are unique and beautiful in your own way, never compare yourself with anyone else, the potential for everything is within you and with God all things are possible.

Please go back and reread the book many times, see what stands out to you, what needs the most attention and set your priorities. Remember to take a holistic approach and to pay attention to all levels, the physical, emotional, mental, energetic and spiritual. Take care of yourself, nourish yourself and believe in yourself. Use radiance as your mantra; see yourself in your mind's eye becoming more and more radiant every day. Live from the spirit within, empower yourself and develop a joyful, passion for life.

About the Author

Maggie Erotokritou is an Ayurvedic health consultant, rebirther, healer, transformational counsellor and Yoga and meditation teacher. She co-directed the Surya Centre for health and healing in Cyprus, founded the Women's Spiritual Network and the Global Spiritual Network on the Internet. She lives and works in Nicosia, Cyprus and also works in London. She gives seminars on health, healing and spiritual development and women's issues.

Her book, Radiant Woman, Every Woman's Guide to Health, Healing and Rejuvenation is based upon many years of personal experience of exploration into different healing modalities including Ayurveda, Esoteric Healing and Rebirthing.

She is deeply interested in the metaphysical and energetic aspects of healing and the study of consciousness and human potential.

For information on individual sessions, seminars and retreats or to order CDs or Yoga videos contact Maggie at
surya@spidernet.com.cy or **MaggieErotokritou@hotmail.com**

For information on the Global Spiritual Network see
www.globalspiritualnetwork.org
To receive the free, daily postings send an email to
surya@spidernet.com.cy

Printed in the United Kingdom
by Lightning Source UK Ltd.
93520